The 4 Day Diet

the 4 Day DIET

Ian K. Smith, M.D.

St. Martin's Press ☙ New York

For Tristé and Dash,

because of you, I am.

Contents

Acknowledgments

As with any book that is fortunate enough to reach the shelves, there are so many people who quietly take their shift on the assembly line, making important contributions to the finished product but receiving little recognition. Unfortunately, most of these unsung "heroes" the author never even gets a chance to meet or know by name. So I want to first acknowledge all of these helpers—whether in the printing plant, art department, or mail room—who really played a big role in making this book become a reality.

My immeasurable gratitude also goes out to Tristé and Dash—my rocks at home, who have graciously tolerated, without a single complaint, my many idiosyncrasies when I'm in "writing mode." My brother, Dana, who always finds a way to push and challenge me and make me better. My cheerleading and constantly thoughtful editor, Elizabeth Beier, and her editorial assistant, Michelle Richter, and the rest of the incredible team at St. Martin's Press—Sally Richardson, Matthew Shear, Steve Cohen, and John Murphy. Pam El for going through the modules of this diet with strength and losing a ton of weight. My personal assistant, Liza Rodriguez, for keeping my life organized. And the thousands of dieters I've worked with over the years, who have taught me as much about weight loss as I've taught them.

Introduction

Losing weight is 80 percent mental and 20 percent physical. Most people spend a great deal of time debating which diet is best and arguing the merits that distinguish one plan from another. Not enough time, however, is spent "training the brain" to take on one of life's toughest journeys—the journey of weight loss. I have worked with thousands of people who have struggled and succeeded in their weight-loss efforts, and I have learned a tremendous amount from their personal experiences. Each person has talked enthusiastically about the most critical piece of their success being something you might find surprising: mental preparation. That is why I've written **THE 4 DAY DIET.** With this book you, too, can share what I've learned—the secrets and the success.

Lack of mental preparation before beginning a weight-loss program is the first and biggest mistake people make before starting on their journey. If you don't get your mind in the right place, it will only work against you, like an anchor dragging behind a boat that is trying to move forward in the water. But pull up that anchor—get your mind ready for what's to come—and that boat will go forward full force.

I have discussed privately and publicly the importance and advantage of mastering the psychology of weight loss. Unfortunately, discussion of the mind's role in getting thin and fit has largely been absent in popular diet books. The mental game is largely ignored because everyone is eager to focus on carbs and calories and exercise regimens. Make no mistake, carbs and calories and exercise are vital to weight loss, but focusing on them before focusing on the mental side of weight loss is like putting the cart ahead of the horse. Your mind will lead you in your battle of the bulge, and your body will execute the mind's strategy. **THE 4 DAY DIET** is a simple, straightforward guide that will help you understand how to set your goals, how to get and stay motivated, and how to resist the temptations that will threaten to derail your journey.

After you've read the first part of **THE 4 DAY DIET,** you will be able to master the mental part of weight loss and be primed to follow the modular eating plan that I have designed in the next section of the book. This eating plan is a unique take on weight loss that has been called "exciting," "simple," and "tremendously effective" by many who have followed it. I have configured **THE 4 DAY DIET** plan in segments of days that allow you to eat a variety of different foods and prevent you from becoming bored and restless, pitfalls that often lead people to abandon those diet programs that ask you to eat the same thing every day. The foods in **THE 4 DAY DIET** eating plan are tasty, inexpensive, and easy to find. Nothing is packaged or fake or full of chemicals. You can easily buy what you need at your local grocery store and get prepared to make small changes that will deliver tremendous results.

As you move forward on your weight-loss journey, remember to utilize all the strategies you learn in the following chapters. If you hit a plateau or find yourself losing the desire to stay on the plan, go back and reread the chapter(s) that will help sharpen your mental focus and psych you up. Refreshing your knowledge and determination will only work to your advantage. On **THE 4 DAY DIET**, you can even have fun. Your mind and body will be constantly evolving as you lose weight, and while the final results are always exciting, you should be equally thrilled by a process that will allow you to do more than just survive but actually feel ALIVE!

Yours in the journey,
Ian K. Smith, M.D.
January 2009

The 4 Day Diet

CHAPTER 1

Sense of Where You Are

START WITH HONESTY

One afternoon I was rummaging through my uncle's vast attic filled with dusty memorabilia, the equivalent of gold to an adventurous teen. I came upon a box that had been pushed into a corner underneath a tangle of dust and cobwebs. Hoping for collectible baseball cards or rare coins, I was disappointed to find a pile of books most of whose titles were so worn I couldn't read them. Those I could read I couldn't understand. But midway through the stack I was drawn to a skinny paperback that featured on its jacket a photograph of a young man dribbling a basketball. The title is what caught my attention: *A Sense of Where You Are*.

A serious athlete myself, I plucked the book from the box, brushed off the dust, and lost myself in its sepia-colored pages. The book was about former presidential candidate, three-term U.S. senator, and one of Princeton University's greatest basketball players, Bill Bradley. From his childhood as a banker's son to his storied career at Princeton, the book told the story of a hardworking, disciplined, intelligent ball player whose tremendous success on the court was largely attributed to his awareness at all times of his position in relationship to the basket, thus the title *A Sense of Where You Are*.

It is this understanding of one's relationship to the ultimate target that became the blueprint for this chapter. Regardless of how fatigued he was, how outmatched athletically, or how fast the pace of the action, Bill Bradley always had that sure sense of where he stood relative to his ultimate goal: scoring a basket. This understanding is also critical for anyone trying to lose weight. Regardless of what's going on in your life, whether it is stress at the job, a busy day of running around with the kids, or traveling for pleasure or business, you must *always* know where you are relative to your goals. It's not about obsessing over your goals but, rather, having them readily present at least in your subconscious so that when you come to one of those proverbial forks in the road, you don't even have to think about the right choice. The right choice becomes a simple reflex of your body.

You will often hear people say that they don't go to the doctor for annual checkups or don't undergo recommended screening tests even though doing so could possibly catch illnesses in their earlier stages when they're most curable. Why don't they want to know what's going on with their bodies? One of the most common and equally mystifying answers is "If there's something going on with me, I don't want to know."

What will best guide your success during **THE 4 DAY DIET** journey is complete honesty and knowing fully what's going on. You will have to face the truths that you discover along the way. Rather than run from these truths or try to bury them, you will learn how to embrace them—starting right now. There are some tough questions that you must answer. Write your answers down in order.

Why are you currently overweight?

Why have previous weight-loss efforts failed?

How does your weight influence your self-esteem/self-image?

What are your strengths related to sticking to a weight-loss program?

What are your weaknesses related to sticking to a weight-loss program?

Without weighing yourself or looking at a Body Mass Index (BMI) chart, how many pounds away do you think you are from your target weight?

Once you've answered these questions, take some time to consider the answers. These answers are critical not only to give context to your current situation but to serve as a springboard moving forward.

Now there is a second set of questions whose answers will give you a better *sense of where you are*. Weigh yourself on a reliable scale, one that is convenient and that you'll be able to use throughout your journey. Once you have the number, use the BMI chart in this chapter to help you answer some of these questions:

What is your current BMI?

What does the chart say is a healthy weight for your height?

What are your bad habits when it comes to exercising/eating right?

What are your good habits when it comes to exercising/eating right?

When was the last time you were at a weight you were happy with?

Keep these answers stored in a place where you won't lose them. You will need to refer to them throughout your weight-loss journey.

WHERE YOU ARE RIGHT NOW: YOUR BMI

Let's get down to work. Every journey needs a starting point, so let's establish yours right now. Your current weight and BMI are a good place to start. According to the Centers for Disease Control, Body Mass Index (BMI) is calculated from a person's weight and height and is a reliable indicator of a person's body fatness. The BMI is used to determine which of four major categories you fit into: underweight, normal, overweight, and obese. Determining which category you fall into is critical because it can help indicate your risk for certain diseases and health conditions.

Your BMI can be calculated or simply found on a BMI chart readily accessible on the Internet. Let's do the calculation here:

$$\frac{\text{WEIGHT (POUNDS)} \quad \text{X} \quad 703}{[\text{height (inches)}]^2}$$

So let's take a man who is 5' 10" (70 inches) and weighs 200 pounds.

$$\frac{200 \ X \ 703}{(70)^2} = 28.7$$

You can also get this number by simply using the BMI chart in the Appendix, page 216. Once you've figured out your BMI, you can look to see which category you fit into.

BMI	WEIGHT STATUS
Below 18.5	Underweight
18.5–24.9	Normal
25–29.9	Overweight
30 and Above	Obese

The man in our sample would be considered overweight according to his BMI. Why does this matter, since he's clearly not obese? His being overweight increases his risk for certain medical conditions and even death.

Diseases and Health Conditions Related to Obesity

Hypertension (high blood pressure)

Dyslipidemia (for example, high LDL cholesterol, low HDL cholesterol, or high levels of triglycerides)

Type 2 diabetes

Coronary heart disease

Stroke

Gallbladder disease

Osteoarthritis

Sleep apnea and respiratory problems

Some cancers (endometrial, breast, and colon)

Source: Centers for Disease Control.

EVERYTHING IS NOT AS IT APPEARS

It's important to distinguish between the medical definition of your weight and the visual interpretation. These can be very different and thus very confusing. You've almost certainly heard the expression "She wears her weight well." This typically refers to people who are overweight but don't look overweight, because they are either very tall or their weight is distributed throughout their body in such a way that no one area looks particularly alarming.

The visual interpretation of weight can be a tricky thing. Just because someone doesn't look overweight doesn't mean that he isn't. Sometimes a person won't appear to be heavy, but then she steps on the scale or calculates her BMI and realizes she is not only overweight, but in some cases obese. I had this happen with a famous plus-size model who insisted that she was "curvy and voluptuous" and not overweight. She was one of the contestants on my show, *Celebrity Fit Club*. Her argument was that she didn't look overweight, that she was full-figured and attractive, and men found her curves irresistible. But her BMI actually pegged her as obese. She not only refused to accept her BMI but even went so far as to suggest the BMI chart was wrong and it didn't apply to her or others like her. In her estimation, the BMI chart had a bias against ethnic women.

The BMI chart is certainly not perfect, but it is the best tool we have to approximate a person's degree of overweight and obesity without a more thorough body fat test in a specialist's office. It was not designed to judge who is beautiful and who isn't. BMI is simply an objective measure. It doesn't know or care about the length of your eyelashes, the color of your skin, or what you do for a living. It simply takes objective measures—your height and your weight—and gives you a number that helps you and your doctor determine your risk for certain diseases.

I have heard many people say, "The chart says that I'm overweight, but I still don't have diabetes or high blood pressure. I'm fine." That might be true—for now. The negative consequences of poor eating habits and lack of physical activity are often not immediate. They slowly add up over time, but be assured that once they reach the critical threshold, adverse health conditions are an inevitability. This is why the medical definition of obesity is better suited than any highly subjective visual interpretation to determine whether weight loss will make you healthier.

UNLOCKING THE MYSTERY OF WHY YOU'RE HERE

No one suddenly wakes up one morning and discovers that she is 30 pounds overweight. There's a reason that the scale is registering the number staring back at you, and it's not because you swallowed a bowling ball before you went to bed last night. Whether it has been years of poor eating, a chronic illness, medications you've taken, a life of too little physical activity, or a slowing of your metabolism, there is a reason or a combination of reasons that you're in this predicament. The first step in making a change is an acknowledgment of where you are and *how* you got there.

We've already figured out your BMI and what your weight status is. This is the "where you are" part. Now it's time to see *how* you arrived at this point in life. This requires more honesty and reflection. Think back to the time when you were at the weight and degree of health that you most enjoyed. Find a quiet place where you won't be distracted, close your eyes, and see an image of yourself at that point in your life—the length of your hair, the shape of your legs, the cut of your jaw. Feel once again what it was like to run up stairs and not be winded. See the size of the clothes that was stamped in the labels. Smell the freshly cut grass of the park you walked in or played softball. Take not only your mind but your entire body back to that point in your life. Once you've been there for five minutes, open your eyes and answer the following questions. You will be completing your own Then/Now chart.

Your Then/Now chart is extremely valuable for your weight-loss success. It provides a road map of not only where you were but also how you got to your current location. Once you've completed this chart, look carefully at the differences between then and now. They can help you pinpoint where and why things changed and your detour began. It can also give you clear directions to get back on course to a healthier weight and better lifestyle. Best of all, the Then/Now chart will prove to you that you had good, strong eating and exercise habits at one point in your life. And if you had them once, you can have them again.

	THEN	NOW
What foods did you eat then that you no longer eat?		
What foods did/do you eat in abundance?		
Three physical activities you enjoy.		
Three hobbies you enjoy.		
People, places, or things that stress you out.		
Where do you get most of your support?		
How do you regard your physical appearance? (No interest, care a little, important, very important.)		
How important is your health? (I don't care, some importance, important, very important.)		
Level of motivation. (None, some, good, very high, excellent.)		

ASSESSING YOUR BODY IMAGE

What you think about yourself really matters. Those thoughts influence your behavior, and that directly impacts what happens to your body. Your body image is the mental picture you have about the way you *think* you look. It involves how you feel about your body's shape, look, overall size, and weight. You might be a normal weight, but if you think you're overweight and unattractive, this could influence the way you eat and exercise. Just the same, if you really are overweight and much larger than what is considered healthy for your height but see yourself as a normal size and weight, then you might be less inclined to make the necessary changes to improve your health risks.

Having a healthy body image also means having a true understanding of whether or not you are at a healthy weight and, if you aren't, an acceptance of the idea that you need to make some behavioral changes.

There are many self-assessment tools available to help you better understand your body image. Here is a quiz that I find simple, direct, and extremely

True or False	I can easily name my favorite body part (other than my hair or eyes).
True or False	I can look at myself in the mirror and see an attractive person looking back.
True or False	I am not preoccupied with when I can and cannot eat.
True or False	I don't need to count calories or fat grams to feel that I am eating healthfully.
True or False	I don't exercise to change my body shape, only to be healthy and happy.
True or False	I never smoke or use drugs to curb my appetite.
True or False	I feel comfortable eating around other people—male or female.
True or False	I don't harm my body when dealing with stress.
True or False	I don't compare the way I look to the way my friends look.
True or False	I don't think I am much bigger or smaller than my friends tell me I am.
True or False	I am comfortable being naked when alone.
True or False	I am comfortable being naked with my partner—even with the lights on.
True or False	I do not feel that I need a sexual partner in order to feel attractive.

The more questions you answered True, the more likely you are to have a positive perception of your body. Keep retaking this quiz over time to gauge your changing body image. Hopefully, the change will be positive. Adapted with permission by the Office of Health Promotion, Villanova University.

useful. It is the Villanova University Body Image Self Quiz. It helps measure how comfortable you are with your body and how accepting you are of yourself.

JOURNALING

You might have heard of a dieting journal, and maybe you've even kept one in the past. Whatever your past experience with journaling, I need you to wipe the slate clean and commit yourself to starting a new one.

Journaling is one of the most effective weight-loss tools you can take on your journey. The cost is minimal—just a notebook and a writing instrument. Keeping an honest journal is another means of helping you maintain a sense of where you are. It's important that you log information that will give you a clear picture of not only what you eat and what type of physical activity you're doing, but also your mood throughout the day. Journaling allows you to identify areas of weakness that can be improved and areas of strength that you should build upon as you go through **THE 4 DAY DIET** program.

Before starting the diet, you should journal for ten days, keeping track of everything and recording as many details about the activity as possible: After these ten days, study your entries and identify your strengths and weaknesses. Some people like to keep journaling and there's nothing wrong with continuing if you'd like to. But for the purposes of beginning an assessment of where you are and gathering information, ten days is enough. Make sure you're as specific as possible in your entries. For example, instead of simply writing that you ate carrots for a snack, write that you ate half a cup of carrots. Instead of writing that you exercised in the morning, write that you performed 30 minutes of cardiovascular exercise of moderate intensity.

This is how a typical **4 DAY DIET** journal entry might look:

Day 1

7 A.M.	1 cup of freshly squeezed orange juice and 1 large banana
7:45 A.M.	35 minutes of cardio (20 minutes treadmill walking—intense; 15 minutes stationary bike)
8:30 A.M.	6 oz of plain low-fat yogurt with fresh sliced strawberries, 1 cup of coffee
11 A.M.	1 small salad topped with nuts and sliced apples, 3 tbsp of low-fat dressing
1:30 P.M.	Chicken sandwich on whole wheat bread, sliced tomato, 1 packet of mayo, 1 slice of provolone cheese, 1 cup of coffee
4 P.M.	15 almonds
7 P.M.	4 oz of salmon, 1 cup of brown rice, 1 serving of broccoli, 1 chocolate brownie
8 P.M.	Walk in the neighborhood—1 mile
9 P.M.	10 crackers, 15 frozen grapes
10 P.M.	Sleep

Comments: Today felt like a good day. My exercise in the morning was strong. I felt a little hungry near the end of my workday, but the snack helped. I realize that I have to keep eating small meals and snacks throughout the day, and that will keep my energy up. The walk after dinner felt good because I felt as if I was burning more calories before going to bed. I'm going to exercise a little longer tomorrow morning.

Work Box

1. Answer the following questions:

   Why are you currently overweight?

   Why have previous weight-loss efforts failed?

   How does your weight influence your self-esteem/self-image?

   What are your strengths related to sticking to a weight-loss program?

   What are your weaknesses related to sticking to a weight-loss program?

   Without weighing yourself or looking at a Body Mass Index (BMI) chart, how many pounds away do you think you are from your target weight?

2. Calculate your BMI and find your category (underweight, normal, overweight, obese).

3. According to the BMI chart, what weight range will give you a healthy BMI?

4. Answer the following questions:

   What are your bad habits when it comes to exercising/eating right?

   What are your good habits when it comes to exercising/eating right?

   When was the last time you were at a weight you were happy with?

5. Complete the Body Image Self Quiz.

CHAPTER 2

Make Realistic Goals

DON'T SET YOURSELF UP FOR FAILURE

A close relative of mine decided that she wanted to make a fortune and get into the real estate game. She had never had much experience with real estate other than purchasing her own houses. Because of her age, lack of experience, and the unpredictable market, I thought it might be tough for her to make that "fortune" she was so sure she'd make, but I encouraged her to follow her dreams.

She studied very hard and earned her broker's license, then promptly joined an established firm and set out to make all those millions that the get-rich books had promised. Her reasoning was simple: "If so many other people could make lots of money selling houses and land, I can, too." Her work ethic and dedication—as they'd been her entire life—were nothing short of intense. She dipped into her savings and began spending relatively large sums of money on advertising, building her own Web site, real estate software, and other accouterments that she had heard were critical for instant success. According to her calculations, she'd make her first million within a couple of years and from there her empire would only grow.

After the first year she analyzed her progress and realized that she was extremely far away from that million-dollar milestone, having sold only four homes during that year. But her spirit and determination were not dampened, and she pushed herself even harder the next year, selling more houses but not enough to land her that million-dollar profit she was certain she'd be able to reach in just two years. It would be an understatement to say that she was disappointed and considered herself a failure for not hitting that million-dollar goal within two years. She had spent most of her savings at this point and was increasingly doubtful whether she'd ever be successful in the real estate business. Over a long Sunday dinner, I gave her my take on the situation.

> You've been extremely successful these two years. You've sold more homes in two years than most new brokers sell in four years. You have a strong stream of referrals, and had you not spent so much money on advertising and some of the non-necessities, you actually would've turned a nice profit. By no stretch of the imagination are you a failure, but the goals you set for yourself and your expectations were so high that failure as you've defined it was practically unavoidable. Unrealistic goals and expectations are a one-direction highway to perceived failure and disappointment.

Many people trying to lose weight find themselves failing not because they aren't losing weight, but because they haven't reached the goals they set for themselves at the beginning of their journey. The vast majority of these goals are not only unrealistic but actually unhealthy due to the demands placed on the body. One of the most common problems: trying to lose too much too fast. Goal setting is the official start of your journey. That is why poor goal setting can lead to disastrous results.

Several studies have shown that the average weight gain for Americans is between 2 and 3 pounds per year. This might surprise many since a 5-pound-a-year figure is often quoted in the popular media. In most cases, weight gain tends to be small and gradual, but it's not until we aren't able to fit into our favorite clothes or someone offhandedly remarks, "Have you put on a few pounds?" that we start realizing it's time to cut back on the calories and start making regular appointments at the gym. When people stop me and say they want to lose weight, the first thing I say is "Are you serious enough, and is this the right time in your life to do it?" The second thing I ask is "How much do you want to lose and over what period of time?"

Eight times out of ten the answer to the second question leaves me shaking my head. How about this conversation I had with one woman who stopped me in the airport a few months ago:

"I want to lose fifty pounds," she said. "I'm tired of carrying around this extra weight."

"I would agree with the fifty as an ultimate goal," I said. "How long do you want to take to lose it?"

She half-closed her eyes the way people do when they're thinking really hard. Then she smiled and said, "I want to lose it in three months."

"Three months?" I said, tightening my brow. "Are you sure?"

She looked at me now with widened eyes. "Can I do it in two months?"

I've had this type of conversation thousands of times, as have most other nutrition and weight-loss experts. People want to lose the weight immediately but they don't take into account that they didn't gain it immediately. If the average person gains only 2 to 3 pounds per year, it typically takes almost ten years before that person looks in the mirror and seriously thinks he needs to do something about the excess weight. What always intrigues me is that given how slowly people let the weight creep up on them, they want it to disappear overnight. This is the *wrong* approach when it comes to safely and effectively losing weight.

Dieters put a great deal of unnecessary pressure on themselves by setting the bar too high. Not only are they setting themselves up to fail, but in many cases they begin resorting to desperate measures that typically involve dangerous eating or exercising habits or taking unsafe supplements. Regardless of what program you are following or what promises the spokespeople for these programs have advertised, *you* need to be in control of *your* goals and the speed at which *you* lose weight. There is vast evidence in the medical literature that says that those who tend to lose the most weight and keep it off the longest are those who lose it gradually and in a healthy manner. This involves making important lifestyle changes rather than short-term adjustments for a quick fix.

SETTING REALISTIC GOALS

So how should you go about setting your realistic goals? One of the easiest ways to do this is something called the S.M.A.R.T. principle, a well-used technique that looks at five characteristics:

Specific

Measurable

Attainable

Realistic

Time Frame

SPECIFIC

It's important to set clearly defined goals. The more specific the goals, the more focused the effort in achieving them. Your goals should be straightforward and easy to understand. It's not effective to simply say, "I want to lose a few pounds." A more directed goal is "I want to lose 30 pounds in six months." Let "what" and "how" guide you in your goal setting. What exactly are you going to do? Lose 30 pounds in six months. How are you going to do it? By making the appropriate dietary and exercise changes recommended by the program I'm following.

MEASURABLE

It's critical that your goal be measurable. This will keep you focused as well as maintain your awareness of where you are in the process. There are several measures when it comes to weight loss, but often we get too stuck on a number. Please don't get me wrong. Yes, the pounds reflected on the scale make a difference, but there are other ways to measure your progress.

The size of the clothing that you fit into can sometimes be the first sign that you're losing weight. I can't count how many times people have said to me, "The scale says that I haven't lost anything, but I can fit into a size eight when just two weeks ago I was a size ten." This is because weight loss isn't always reflected in numbers but is often reflected in the changing size and shape of our body. So it's completely fine to set your dress or waist size as a goal. Many people who find themselves stalled on the scale can become discouraged by the lack of results, but if they had losing a dress or pant size as a benchmark for success, they'd realize progress was still being made and remain optimistic and motivated. Look for positive reinforcement everywhere, whether it's a colleague complimenting how great you look or your doctor noting how the weight loss has improved your blood pressure, cholesterol levels, diabetes, or other health indicators. Basing success strictly on the number on the scale is not taking into account the true complexity of body transformation.

Weight loss can be a complicated process that involves more than just a reduction in pounds. The body is composed of many tissue types, including fat, muscle, bones, ligaments, and tendons. Water is the biggest component of our weight—according to some estimates as much as 60 to 70 percent. Water and all these tissues are constantly changing, especially as we lose weight. Sometimes one might lose fat but also start gaining muscle as a result of resistance training (lifting weights). There could also be water loss or gain depending on the amount of liquids you drink and whether your body has a tendency to hold on to fluids or readily eliminate them. Depending on when you step on the scale, it's virtually impossible to know what's happening inside your body with respect to water balance and the various tissues that contribute to your overall weight.

Some people actually monitor their weight-loss progress by regularly taking body fat measurements. This is my least favorite method because how one loses weight from the different body tissues is unpredictable at best, especially when it comes to body fat percentage. There's also another major flaw with this technique: consistent accuracy. Taking reliable and accurate body fat measurements can be a rigorous process, and it's easy to make errors even with dedicated effort and experience. If you are someone who really worries about body fat percentage and you're determined to use that as your measurement of progress, it's imperative that you choose the same method each time and take the measurements from the same body parts.

ATTAINABLE

It makes no sense to set a goal that you can't reach. Being able to attain a goal makes both failure and success honest. A goal beyond reach means that the failure associated with not reaching it is false. Don't misinterpret this point to mean that I'm suggesting you make the goal easy. The goal should be challenging but attainable. When the target is out of reach, the pursuer will inevitably be discouraged and could easily give up on the mission.

An unattainable goal can also lead to unhealthy behaviors. Fasting or severely restricting your calorie intake over a long period of time can be extremely dangerous and in fact actually counterproductive when it comes to weight loss. When your body isn't properly nourished and isn't receiving enough calories to perform the daily functions of life, it automatically switches into conservation or starvation mode. In starvation mode, the body holds on to every calorie it takes in and also tries to hold on to the fat stores because it doesn't know when it will see its next decent meal. This is exactly what you *don't* want to happen when trying to lose weight.

Set a goal that is going to require dedication, hard work, and perseverance. A goal that's too easy to attain might mean that you're not asking enough of yourself and have set the bar too low. Look at it like this: Have you ever been the weight you want to achieve? If the answer is no, then it's unlikely you will reach that weight and be able to stay there over the long term. If the answer is yes but not for the last ten or fifteen years, then it's possible you could reach this goal, but it will require discipline and patience to achieve it because your metabolism has likely slowed and your body has grown accustomed to the heavier weight. What you weighed in high school is unlikely to be what you'll be able to attain and maintain in adulthood, so keep this in mind when you're setting the goal.

REALISTIC

Realism is the close cousin of attainability. Your goal must be something that you're able to work toward given a reasonable degree of difficulty. It is unrealistic to pick up a tennis racket for the first time and expect to be talented enough to qualify for Wimbledon within the next two years. Losing 30 pounds in two months because you're going on vacation and want to look your best in a bathing suit is unrealistic. I know people who have been able to meet that goal, but those people are rare.

Your goal must be something that you're willing to work hard to reach, but it must also be attainable. When a goal is unrealistic, there's a greater likelihood that you will realize long before you've even come close to the goal that it's too tough, leading to discouragement and your eventually giving up. The success of your program could depend more than you think on how realistic a goal you set for yourself.

TIME FRAME

It's important for your goal to be set within a time frame. Having your goal linked to a time clock gives it a sense of urgency and direction. Simply saying you want to lose 20 pounds doesn't move you into action. You could start today . . . or tomorrow . . . or when things slow down at work. But when you say that you want to lose 20 pounds in four months, then your goal and actions to reach that goal come with some urgency. It's customary for a dieter to aim for an average weight loss of one to two pounds per week. This would be a commendable success.

SMALLER GOALS ADD UP TO THE BIG GOAL

The way you structure your ultimate goal can make a big difference. What's important is not simply to have the ultimate big goal but to break up that goal into smaller goals or milestones. This prevents you from being overwhelmed by the magnitude of the big goal. Let's say you want to lose 45 pounds. That can be an overpowering number if you just think how far you have to go and how long it could take to reach it. But if you think about losing 6 pounds, then 8 pounds, and then 4 pounds, all the way to 45 pounds, it seems like something you can accomplish. This is what marathoners and other long-distance runners do masterfully. Instead of thinking about the entire 26.2 miles they have to run, they break the race into smaller segments. For each segment they set an individual goal for the time they want to complete it in. This is tremendously effective not just strategically but also from a psychological standpoint. It can be daunting to stand at the start line and think about 26.2 long miles and the hundreds of runners you're competing against to finish first. But if you break up the 26.2 miles into 3- or 4-mile segments, your mind sees the race as a series of piece-of-cake smaller races rather than a long, grueling one.

MORE THAN THE SCALE

So much of our focus is on the number—how much we weigh when we step on the scale. For many it can become an obsession, and it's when your focus reaches this level of zeal that you have created a problem. That is why it's important before you start a program that you set other goals that have nothing to do with the scale. These other goals should keep you moving toward the big goal, but they should be different enough to draw attention away temporarily from the finish line.

The list of other goals you might set is practically infinite. Your list might include the following:

- Run a mile in under 9 minutes
- Drop two dress sizes
- Lower your blood pressure
- Eat at least five servings of fruits and vegetables each day
- Do some form of exercise five days a week
- Lower your cholesterol level
- Convince at least one other person to make life changes to improve health
- Be able to do a consecutive 35 minutes of cardiovascular exercise
- Love what you see in the mirror and accept your body's changes

I suggest starting out with at least three of these alternate goals. Try to be specific about when you'd like to reach the goal. For example, let's say you want to run a mile in under 9 minutes but currently are running a 12-minute mile. You might want to give yourself 3 months to reach this goal. Treat these alternate goals as you do the big goal. Be specific about what you want to accomplish and when you want to accomplish it. Don't just regard these goals as incidental landmarks you just happen to pass as you journey toward the ultimate goal, but instead place significant value on reaching them. They not only represent improvement but affirm that you are making progress.

As you attain your alternate goals, make sure you set new ones. Imagine that you are a sightseer on a mission to visit the Eiffel Tower in Paris and ride to the top to enjoy that famous vantage point over the City of Lights. You could simply get in a cab and have the driver take you directly to the tower and ignore everything else the city has to offer. But the more rewarding journey might be one that includes stopping at the Louvre, visiting Notre Dame, touring the Grand Palais, and passing underneath the Arc de Triomphe. These landmarks are significant in their own right, even if they may not have the international popularity of the Eiffel Tower. You would leave Paris with a more enriched experience having visited these other landmarks in addition to reaching the top of the tower. You enrich your journey by achieving the smaller milestones along the way to your ultimate goal. Every single one you can check off your list will make you feel great.

UPDATE YOUR GOAL

Goals should not be fixed targets but should be regarded as dynamic. As human beings we are constantly evolving, adapting to our environment and the life experiences from which we constantly learn. It's important to start off with an ultimate goal in mind, but you should also be prepared to *adjust* this big goal along the course of your journey. Just as life can be unpredictable, so can weight loss and all the factors that can work either to your advantage or disadvantage.

Recently I had the pleasure of working with a famous actress who I'll call BL. She was in a twelve-week weight-loss competition and older than all the others she was competing against. We set a twelve-week goal of 20 pounds, which was ambitious considering that she was not physically active and only needed to lose approximately 25 pounds to achieve a healthy BMI. Because she was not extremely overweight—75 pounds or more—she would have to work hard to lose such a significant amount of weight in such a short period of time. Typically, the closer you are to your goal weight, the more difficult it is to lose those extra pounds.

BL was skeptical about the goal I had set. She had been on several diets recently and had lost and gained weight like other yo-yo dieters. BL was not a fan of exercise and knew that this would be to her disadvantage since regular exercise would accelerate her weight-loss efforts. But despite her reservations, BL was a good sport, accepted the goal, and made a commitment to work her hardest to achieve it.

BL's first two weeks were phenomenal. I put her on a detox plan, and she lost a remarkable 11 pounds. That meant she needed to lose only 9 pounds in ten weeks to hit her goal, an average of less than a pound a week. I was confident she would do it, especially since she had an entirely different attitude two weeks in than when she started. Now that she had experienced some success, she was enthusiastic about experiencing more. **Success begets success.** Two weeks went by, and BL lost another 3 pounds. Her weight loss was consistent and admirable.

The sixth week she weighed in and had lost another 4 pounds, which meant she was down 18 pounds in just half the time we had set for her to reach her goal. She was winning the contest easily, and her enthusiasm for the diet program and even the exercise portion (which she detested in the beginning) was miraculous to watch. She stood before the other competitors and proclaimed that she was voluntarily changing her goal. She was feeling so good and was so pleased with the results of the diet program that she wanted to lose 30 pounds instead of the original 20. I enjoyed seeing BL's transformation from a skeptical participant to a leader. I also enjoyed watching the others become inspired by her example. Not only did she win the competition by a landslide, but she ended up losing 34 pounds in twelve weeks. What was more remarkable than the number was that she had made important lifestyle changes; she was eating better foods and incorporating the once-dreaded exercise into her normal routine. BL ended the competition proclaiming how much she now enjoyed exercising and couldn't imagine not doing it for the rest of her life.

Goals can be raised or lowered as one moves along the weight-loss journey. There are legitimate reasons that your goal can go either way. BL had good reasons to increase her goal, but others might find that the first goal they set was too ambitious or they encounter temporary setbacks such as injury or being placed on medications (such as steroids, antidepressants, or blood pressure medications) that unfortunately cause weight gain. You must determine what goal is achievable, safe, and satisfying, and this can change as you actually engage in the process of losing weight. I believe everyone should take a closer look at their goal at each quarter mark. Let's say you have set a goal of 40 pounds in twelve months. Every quarter—or third month—you should look at where you are in relation to achieving your goal and whether you think you're ahead of schedule or behind. You may choose to keep the goal where it is or alter it, but keeping tabs on your progress and reevaluating the goal throughout the journey is essential.

SETTING YOUR GOALS

Now that you understand the importance of appropriate goal setting, it's time to get to work. While the following strategy is one that I have used successfully for years and it has helped thousands, remember that goal setting is as personal as choosing the furniture in your house and the color you want to paint your walls. You ultimately have to make the decision, but you can use my strategy as a guideline.

FIGURING OUT THE ULTIMATE GOAL: *THE FAT SMASH* GOAL SETTER

A. I believe everyone should strive to be at a healthy weight. It doesn't mean you'll necessarily get there, but if you don't set it as a goal, you'll certainly never make it. Your Body Mass Index (BMI) is the best marker for assessing the healthy weight range in which you want to fall, so figure out your BMI (see Chapter 1) and what the healthy weight range is for your height. For the purpose of instruction I'm going to choose a forty-year-old, 5-foot 4-inch woman who weighs 180 pounds. According to the BMI chart (see Appendix), her current BMI is 30.9, which means she is obese. Her target healthy weight range for her height—according to the BMI chart—is between 107 and 144 pounds. This means she can choose a number anywhere in that range and be considered at a healthy weight when she achieves it. Let's say she chooses 135 pounds, which means a total weight loss of 45 pounds. Achieving her goal would give her a healthy BMI of 23.2.

B. Let's figure out the length of time it would probably take for her to lose 45 pounds. Fair weight loss is an average of 0–1 pound per week. Good weight loss is an average of 1–2 pounds per week. Excellent results would be an average of 2–3 pounds per week. Losing more than 3 pounds on a weekly basis could be losing weight too fast, which can be unhealthy depending on how you lost the weight. How do you decide which category suits you? The eight FAT SMASH GOAL SETTER questions below will help. Our sample dieter's answers are in parentheses.

1. When you've lost weight in the past, how many pounds on average did you lose per week? (One.)
2. Are you willing to exercise at least four days a week for 45 minutes each session? (No. I can only do three days a week.)
3. Do you see yourself struggling with eating the foods your program recommends? (Yes, because I don't like some of them, so I know I'll cheat a little.)
4. How old are you? (Forty.)
5. Will you be able to focus on your weight loss, or are there major life stressors on the horizon? (I will be able to focus completely.)
6. Do you have any medical conditions or are you taking any medications that will slow your weight-loss efforts? (No.)
7. How would you assess your willpower to stick to the program—poor, fair, good, very good, or excellent? (Fair.)

The key to valuing answers is as follows:

Question	Answers	Points
1.	0–1 pound	0.5
	1–2 pounds	1.0
	2–3 pounds	1.5
	3–4 pounds	2
2.	1 day	−1
	2 days	0
	3 days	1

Question	Answers	Points
	4 days	2
	5 days	3
3.	Yes	0
	No	2
4.	30 or more	0
	Under 30	2
5.	Full focus	2
	Good focus but some distraction	1
	Many distractions (trouble at work, relationship problems, money issues)	0
6.	Yes to either one	−1
	No	2
7.	Yes	2
	No	0
8.	Poor	−1
	Fair	0
	Good	1
	Very good	1.5
	Excellent	2

(continued)

The point totals would put you in the following weight-loss categories:

Point Totals	Weight Loss Category
−2.5–6.5	Fair
6.6–13	Good
14–17	Excellent
6.5>–<13	Good
13≥–≤17	Excellent

Our sample dieter has a point total of 7.5, which means she can expect good weight loss—an average of 1–2 pounds per week, if the conditions and plan surrounding her diet stay the same. For the sake of our example, let's say she can lose 1.5 pounds a week. A goal of 45 pounds total weight loss means it would take thirty weeks for her to reach her goal.

45 POUNDS ÷ 1.5 POUNDS PER WEEK = 30 WEEKS

Now for the final calculation. Because no one is perfect and anyone losing weight will hit plateaus and difficult periods, we add a comfort factor—some extra time—to give a cushion.

Multiply the number of weeks you've already calculated by 30 percent:
30 weeks × .30 = 9 weeks (the comfort factor)

Now add the comfort factor to the previously calculated number of weeks:
30 weeks + 9 weeks = 39 weeks

Our sample dieter should set this goal: lose 45 pounds in 39 weeks

Work Box

ESTABLISH YOUR ULTIMATE GOAL

(Use the goal-setting exercise in this chapter.)

Total Weight Loss _____

Number of Weeks _____

SET YOUR THREE ALTERNATE GOALS:

_____

_____

_____

BONUS

S.M.A.R.T.E.R. TIMING

Losing weight isn't just about what you eat or how much you eat. It can depend on *when* you eat. Most people don't understand how important timing is to a weight-loss program. The best eating model to demonstrate this is the French one. I've been to France several times, and one of the first things I noticed—after the spectacular architecture—is how everyone seems to be eating at all times of the day. The little bistros and cafés are open throughout the day and into the night. Americans are accustomed to eating at set hours. Most of our restaurants have specific breakfast, lunch, and dinner hours. Sure, we have diners that are open throughout the day, but diners aren't located in every neighborhood.

The French eat every few hours, but I don't mean sitting down to a five-course meal where they load up on a thousand calories at one sitting. They eat lightly, and they eat often, and they do less snacking on those extra calories. Now that we better understand nutrition and the body's response to food, we understand how advantageous this pattern of eating is in preventing significant weight gain. In America we have been raised on the concept of "three square meals a day" as well as "eating everything on your plate!" At the risk of sounding like a cultural heretic, these traditional beliefs are not doing any good for our waistlines. Lighter and more frequent meals are overwhelmingly advantageous for several reasons, including these:

• Fewer cravings between meals (suppresses appetite)
• Better stabilized blood sugars (fewer spikes)
• Even distribution of calories throughout the day
• Reduction of cortisol levels (high levels of the hormone cortisol are associated with abdominal fat)

Calories, exercise, and the glycemic index of foods (see Chapter 3) still matter when trying to lose weight. However, the timing of your meals and snacks can give you a significant edge in your quest for faster, more effective weight loss. Eating more frequently is believed to increase the hormone leptin in your blood. Leptin has been classified as an appetite suppressant. The reasoning goes that the higher the levels of leptin in your blood, the less likely you are to be hungry.

Stabilizing your blood sugars is important as it relates to the hormone insulin. Insulin is used by the body to sweep glucose (sugar) into the body's cells. The more regular your blood sugar levels are, the more regular your insulin levels and the more evenly you absorb sugars into your cells. If you have spikes in your blood sugars, the result will be an inappropriate release of insulin, which ultimately can cause too much sugar to be absorbed and the creation of fat. (See Chapter 3 for more on this and the glycemic index.)

Distributing your calories evenly throughout the day means your body has a better chance of burning them away. Large meals that are full of calories can present difficulties for your body's metabolism (the body's calorie-burning furnace) and lead to weight gain. This even calorie distribution also means you won't be hungry, one of the major triggers for overeating.

The stress hormone cortisol is released by our adrenal glands and is involved in several bodily functions including: proper glucose metabolism, regulation of blood pressure, release of insulin, the body's inflammatory response to injury, and immune system function. It's called the *stress* hormone because it is secreted for many reasons, including when the body is in the "fight or flight" response mode to stress. High cortisol levels have been associated with abdominal fat, so many scientists believe that by lowering your cortisol levels you can prevent the increase in abdominal fat.

Remember that when you're eating more meals (and snacks) each day, it's important that these meals be smaller or you will simply end up overeating and hurting your weight-loss efforts. Try to be as consistent as possible with the timing of your meals so that your body can get into a rhythm and grow accustomed to its regular flow of energy. Some people might find it difficult to eat several times a day because of a busy schedule or accommodating others in the family, but planning your meals just the way you would a meeting roster, an afternoon of errands, or anything else could make it much easier to fit everything into your day.

CHAPTER 3

Activate Your Motivational Engines

Imagine a complete stranger walking up to you with a twenty-dollar bill, handing it over, and saying, "Please buy me a great lunch that I will enjoy and never forget." If you accept the challenge, your next move might be to ask a series of questions: What kind of food do you like? Do you eat meat? Do you have any food allergies? What foods do you dislike? Would you like a hot or cold meal? There are many other questions you could ask to try to figure out what type of lunch would make this stranger happy.

Why do you need to ask all these questions? Because you don't know this person, and without some type of guidance, it's highly unlikely that you will be able to pick a meal that the person "will enjoy and never forget."

I find myself in a similar situation when people e-mail me or stop me in airports and say, "Dr. Ian, I want to lose weight and I want to follow your diet, but I need motivation. Can you motivate me?" My response is automatic: "I don't know how to motivate someone I don't know."

There is no such thing as a one-size-fits-all strategy when it comes to motivating dieters. You might be motivated to lose weight because you don't want to suffer from heart disease the way your father did. Your friend might be motivated to lose weight because she wants to fit into a pair of jeans she hasn't worn in a year. Your cousin might be motivated to lose weight by her desire to take better control of her diabetes and eventually lower her blood sugar levels so that she no longer requires daily diabetic medications. There is an infinite number of reasons that people are motivated to start a weight-loss program and stick to it. This is why it's so difficult to prescribe a motivational strategy for strangers. Unless you know the person, how would you know what gets him going?

The best way to be motivated and stay motivated is to discover those motivating factors yourself. I've worked with thousands of people who have taken their own weight-loss journeys and discussed with them my concept of a *motivational engine*. Each of us has a motivational engine buried in our core. Some of us are familiar with our engine and can access it as needed. Others have found their engine in the past, but after not using it for a period of time, they have to discover it again. Then there are those very few people who have never found their motivational engine and have spent most of their lives doing whatever comes and allowing circumstances to dictate their lives.

Finding your motivational engine is key to succeeding at any plan or any diet. You may think you know yourself, but as you explore "what makes you tick," you'll learn new things about yourself. Below are a few strategies that you can use to find your motivational engine.

FOUR MOTIVATIONAL QUESTIONS

1. Name three things you've accomplished in life that have made you proud.
2. In the past when you've tried to accomplish something difficult and the odds were stacked against you, what inspired you to continue and eventually succeed?
3. If you faced a physical challenge sometime in your life (finishing a race while exhausted; carrying bags of groceries even when your hands and arms were begging you to put the groceries down; walking a long distance under tough weather conditions but not giving up) or have gone the extra distance such as spending long hours studying to pass a test or finishing a work assignment, what did you mentally focus on to get you through the pain and discomfort and the temptation to quit?
4. Is there someone in your life you would do almost anything for?

ANALYZE YOUR ANSWERS

Take a close look at your answer to question 1. Consider the three accomplishments individually. What was it that helped you stay focused and work hard to complete the tasks that had been set before you? One of my proudest accomplishments was graduating from medical school. The rigorous four years of training were anything but easy, and there were plenty of nights that I was either too tired to study or too discouraged because while I was stuck in the library reading about muscles and tissues, other university students were having a good time partying or going to the movies. What allowed me to study through the fatigue and keep my head in the books even as I heard the merry sound of revelers drifting through the windows of the library? Answer: the image of one day walking across that graduation stage and having the dean hand me my medical school diploma. That simple image, an act that would last no more than eight seconds from the time I walked up the steps on one side of the stage to the time I descended the other side, was all I needed. My hunger for those eight seconds and the perceived satisfaction they would bring to my life was enough to keep me focused and shut out the distractions that might prevent the dream from becoming a reality. Those eight seconds constituted a motivational engine.

Now look at your answer to question 2. It's likely that at some point in your life you've succeeded against the odds. What was it that gave you the strength to persevere and remain determined to succeed? I will never forget reading about the amazing story of Irma Galvan, a mother of four whose husband was murdered in a robbery in Houston, Texas. She was working at a furniture store at the time and was suddenly left to raise four boys by herself. Galvan said that due to the tragic death of her husband, "all of a sudden we were left with no insurance and no future." To make matters even worse, she lost her job after twenty-eight years. So she decided to open a taco stand to serve lunch to area workers on a rundown corner in the dilapidated warehouse district that others were fleeing in droves.

Tenacity, courage, and hope helped her grow the business slowly into a full-fledged, thriving restaurant—Irma's Mexican Restaurant, an eatery that attracts everyone from local celebrities to downtown business customers who years ago never would have traveled into this part of the city. The neighborhood has undergone a great economic boon with new development, and Galvan now owns half the block where her taco stand once stood. Galvan's motivation to beat the odds was the desire to make a better life for her family. She was also *determined* not to quit.

> When I started my business, it never entered my mind to quit. I couldn't quit. If I quit, I would always regret not going and doing what I wanted to do. You have to keep going. You cannot go back and say, "I failed," because it will haunt you forever. When I do a job, I want to give it 100 percent. I give it all I have.

Take whatever it was that helped you beat the odds in your life the way Galvan did, and harness the power of that motivation to help you along your weight-loss journey.

Your answer to question 3 might be the perfect motivational source to help you stay committed to the physical portion of your program. Many people are unable or unwilling to follow the exercise portion of a weight-loss program. This is unfortunate since studies repeatedly show that those who lose the most weight and keep it off the longest are those who not only change their dietary habits but also engage in regular physical activity.

At some point in your life you've probably had to endure some type of physical discomfort to complete a task. It is also likely that despite your body's desire to quit, your mind pulled you through. What did you focus on while completing your task? Some athletes in grueling competitions talk about envisioning the faces of their children as inspiration. What feeling did you focus on to distract you from the immediate discomfort? When I was a teenager, I played football. I remember the wind sprints at the end of practice were always so tough that I felt as if my body was going to suddenly collapse on the field. (Thankfully, that never actually happened.) I would often think about sitting on the grass with my helmet off and ice cold water sliding down the back of my throat. That single simple thought successfully distracted me from the physical pain of the running. Do you have a similar experience? Try to use that when your determination sags.

Your answer to question 4 can be extremely telling. The person you've identified in this answer could be your "weight-loss muse," similar to the muses that writers use to inspire them as they create their stories or poems. I remember that as a child when there was something difficult we had to accomplish, whether taking bad-tasting medicine, walking a long distance in the summer, or braving the cold during the winter, the older children used to tell us, "Do it for someone you really love. Think about how proud they would be of you." It sounds too easy, but the motivational impact was quite powerful. Sometimes forming a mental image of your muse or connecting your action to the muse can provide just enough of a motivational edge to get you over the hump.

AFFIRMATIONS

I'm always interested in where successful people find their motivation and how they are able to sustain it once they've found success. One common thread that weaves through the lives of many success stories is the philosophy of positive thinking. I used to think the concept of positive thinking was nothing more than one of those ambiguous concepts people pay hundreds of dollars to hear motivational speakers throw around at overcrowded seminars. But then I met a Fortune 500 CEO who told me how he had made the decision earlier in his career to incorporate positive thinking in his life and shut out the negativity that always seemed to be lurking around the corner. He decided to see the good in everything and use that to make difficult situations not only tolerable but valuable experiences that yielded important lessons. He also talked about his daily regimen of affirmations—positive assertions—that he repeated to himself every day, sometimes in the morning when he woke up or quietly in his head in the middle of board meetings. His assertions became his reality, and he just kept reminding himself of things until they were not just something he said and thought but a part of who he was.

Create your own affirmations to bolster what you're trying to accomplish. Below are some examples of affirmations that might support someone trying to lose weight.

I can lose weight and keep it off.

I can make myself and my body priorities in my life.

I can open my mind to making changes in my life.

I can withstand some pain to bring about gain.

I can resist the temptations of sweets.

I can see this program through to the end.

Your affirmations can be as long as you'd like them to be, though I suggest making them succinct and memorable. Write each affirmation on an index card—one per card. You might even make several sets of cards so that you can keep one set at work, one at home, and one in your purse or briefcase. Start by reading your affirmations once a day. Find a quiet place where you won't be distracted and then hold the card at arm's length. As you read the affirmation, make sure you focus on the words and form a visual image that represents the goal of the affirmation. Repetition is critical, so make sure you set aside enough time every day to go through your affirmation ritual. For consistency, try to have your session as close to the same time as possible and in the same place every day. For example, you might sit on the edge of your bed every morning after you wake up and read your affirmations.

Once the affirmations have been imprinted in your brain and you have settled on the visual image that goes with each affirmation, you might not need to read them anymore. Instead, just quietly repeat them from memory. Even if you're on vacation or a business trip, make sure you find the time and a place to do your affirmations.

MOTIVATION TO START A PROGRAM

You want to start a program. You know what you need to do to start a program. But you find yourself always putting off your start until tomorrow. The most common motivational question is "How do I get motivated to begin a program?" Some people will never start a program, because they can't effectively combine reason with ambition to create combustion. You first must have a reason to lose weight and believe in the seriousness of that reason. Many people think they have a reason, but it's a weak reason. "I want to lose weight because the cashier at my local store asked me if I had put on a few pounds." This doesn't rank as a powerful reason for wanting to lose weight. Basing your decision to start a program on that exchange could mean the spark will never be big enough to get you going.

Ambition is the other part of this combustible equation. It's possible that you have a good reason to lose weight—your doctor has told you that you're pre-diabetic, and if you don't lose weight, you're going to need medications—but if you don't have the ambition, that inner drive to act, then the best reason in the world will be of no use. Ambition is not something that can be taught. It's a state of mind and a resolve that one must develop. I like to associate ambition with passion, because your feelings must be strong enough to goad you to action.

As you search for your "combustible equation," some motivators might spur you on.

TYPICAL MOTIVATORS

Motivational engines can be extremely personal and unique, so it's virtually im-possible to find motivational triggers that are universally effective. But after spending years helping tens of thousands of people lose weight and find success, I have learned that many of the common triggers can be put into a few large groups. These groups are health benefits, emotions, financial/material gains, peer pressure, success/competitiveness, self-esteem, physical/aesthetic, and health benefits.

Read the descriptions below and see if any of them apply to you. It's pos-sible that some of these triggers have worked for you in the past, and there's a good chance they will work for you again.

HEALTH BENEFITS

Considering the attention that has been given to the world's obesity crisis, it would be difficult to find someone who doesn't know about the risks and dan-gers that are posed by being overweight and obesity. Type 2 diabetes, high blood pressure, stroke, heart disease, and even some forms of cancer are all potential medical complications of obesity. Many people have family mem-bers who were overweight and either suffered greatly from these complica-tions or died from them. Because they witnessed a loved one struggle with the consequences of an unhealthy lifestyle, they are motivated to avoid a similar path of poor decision making and its consequences.

The desire to either become healthy or prevent disease can be extremely powerful and enough of a motivator to get some dieters committed for the long term. Look at how many emotions this can envelop: fear of getting sick, sadness for being in danger, hope that they will not suffer a similar fate as others, and anger at a loved one for knowing they could have avoided the pain of illness had they changed certain behaviors.

EMOTIONS

This might be one of the most common motivational triggers for people trying to lose weight. People report a broad range of emotions when asked how they were able to start a program and finish it. Desire, pain, fear, anger, happiness, shame, anxiety, disgust, sadness, hope, and despair are common emotions that are often discussed when it comes to dieting motivation. Motivational coaches are quick to encourage people to tap into their "emotional being" and allow their deep feelings to serve as prods to success.

It's not uncommon for people to talk about their emotions when asked about the specific turning point when they were able to make major changes in their life: "I went shopping for a new suit, and I had gained so much weight in my waist that I had to find something that was two sizes bigger than what I had been wearing the last five years. I was so disgusted with myself that I vowed to make a change in my life." Others have expressed fear: "I was so afraid that one day I'd be walking up a flight of stairs and my heart would just give out from carrying so much weight. Who would care for my little children if I died?"

Emotional motivation is personal, and you can own it. You can tap into it at will and create a physiologic response inside your body that guides you in your decision making and gives you the strength to stick it out through the tough times or resist the urge to do those things that will hinder your progress.

FINANCIAL/MATERIAL GAIN

I've met plenty of people and read many stories about people who were unsuccessful at weight loss in the past or unwilling to put forth the effort but have suddenly jumped into the fight and changed their eating habits and activity levels. While it always seems like the "pure" motivation should be improving one's health and preventing the onset of weight-related medical complications, the truth is that for many this alone is not enough to get them off the couch and out of the cookie jar. They do it because they stand to gain financially or even win a prize or fame as seen on the popular TV weight-loss shows.

Contests that reward weight loss with cash or prizes are very successful for many who otherwise would have put off their weight-loss efforts for "tomorrow." Some groups form friendly competitions at the office where the participants contribute to a cash pool and the winner or winners are rewarded according to their degree of success. Even reality television has become a motivator as people compete to win not only hundreds of thousands of dollars but a chance at fame, even if in most cases it proves to be fleeting.

I've met couples where one spouse has offered a certain amount of money per pound lost or a big prize for reaching a goal weight. I've heard of jewelry, cars, clothes, and more that have been used to encourage weight loss within families. For some this is just the incentive they need to get going and keep going. If this is what works for you, go for it.

PEER PRESSURE

A study recently appeared in *The New England Journal of Medicine* that showed weight gain could be "contagious" within a close circle of friends. But it showed that weight *loss* could be "contagious," too. People tend to follow the behaviors of their peer group. By the time we reach adulthood, peer pressure is certainly not a new concept. From the first day we stepped into our nursery school or kindergarten class, we were open targets for peer pressure. It's a regular part of our socialization experience, and it exists throughout our lives regardless of age.

Some who have found the determination to get on a program attribute it to their friends or coworkers. It is not uncommon to hear "Everyone at the office was going on a diet and losing weight, so I figured why shouldn't I?" One scenario that I always find interesting concerns weddings. Everyone wants to look good for a wedding, especially the bridesmaids. Bridesmaids will typically have their fittings together or in front of the bride, and women will suddenly get serious because they don't want to look out of place when everyone else is slimming down to look their best.

SUCCESS/COMPETITIVENESS

Sometimes people are motivated because they want to prove a point. Often an offhand statement about someone's appearance or weight starts the ball in motion. There are times when the banter can go as far as a challenge being issued: "I bet any amount of money you can't start a diet and see it to the end. You've never been able to do it before." For many, losing weight is a challenge, and like other challenges, they want to overcome it. Some people are truly addicted to success. They want to lose the weight simply because they want to show themselves and/or others that like everything else in their life, they can be successful at this, too.

Some view dieting as a test, another obstacle to overcome on their journey to success. They understand the health benefits of losing weight, but what really keeps their fire burning is the deep-seated desire to win. People who tend to be goal-oriented and task-driven look at weight loss as one more feat they need to accomplish in a long line of challenges that comprise life.

SELF-ESTEEM

Pride can be one of the biggest motivators, especially when it's attached to one's self-esteem. Most people want to feel good about themselves. We want to be proud of who we are and what we represent. Being overweight and made fun of or ostracized can foster the opposite feeling. Not only do we feel left out, but we feel bad about ourselves, embarrassed, ashamed, and depressed. Unless you're strong-willed and supremely confident, the opinions and actions of others can eventually change how you view yourself.

The desire to respect yourself and feel proud about the person you are can be extremely powerful and motivating. It sounds corny, but sometimes a long, honest look in the mirror can tap into something underneath the surface and spark the inner voice that calmly says, "C'mon, you can do better than this."

PHYSICAL / AESTHETIC

Vanity is part of all of us, and that's not a bad thing. The great nineteenth-century French novelist Gustave Flaubert once said, "I have come to have the firm conviction that vanity is the basis of everything and finally that what one calls conscience is only inner vanity." It's no mystery that many people want to lose weight just because they want to look better. People will often send me e-mails asking for urgent advice because they need to lose weight before going on vacation, to the beach, a reunion, or some other event where they want to impress others with their physical appearance.

Many health experts express concern when people say their motivation for losing weight is to improve their physical appearance. They're worried that someone whose dominant motivation is skin deep won't be able to stick to it. This motivational trigger has a high risk of being temporary, but I believe that for many, vanity is at least a start. Once they start losing weight, looking better, and feeling better, they might discover other sources of motivation that will sustain their weight loss.

SOCIAL BENEFITS

It's easier being thin than fat in this world. While our waistlines are universally expanding, there still are serious stigma attached to being fat. Several studies have documented all types of discrimination faced by overweight people, in everything from job disparities to treatment in hospitals. It has been documented that larger people are less likely to be chosen for jobs when competing against others who are at a healthier weight.

MOTIVATION TO STICK WITH A PROGRAM

You've been on a program for some time, the results are not what you had hoped, and now you're discouraged. You'd rather quit than continuously get on the scale and see a number that indicates, despite all your efforts, that you're failing. The second most common motivational question is "How do I *keep* going once I've started a program?"

Early acknowledgments are important for later success. Most people give up or quit a program because they weren't honest about what awaited them before they started the journey. Regardless of how hard you work or how focused you are on doing the "right" thing, there will be times during your journey that you will be disappointed. This disappointment, whether it's because you've hit a plateau and the weight isn't coming off the way it once was or you're not getting the results you expected from the onset, is completely normal and should not discourage you from continuing your program.

You *must* believe not only in the program you're following but in your own ability to deliver. A shaky belief in either one will not serve you well and will make you vulnerable to impulsive decisions such as quitting the program or participating—even if briefly—in behaviors that fall outside the program's guidelines. Like anything else in life, there are ups and downs in weight loss and several variables at play that determine your short-term and long-term success. Having a strong belief system in place is akin to building the strongest possible foundation for a house. Only catastrophic and unpreventable circumstances can overwhelm a rock-solid foundation.

Finding success—even small success—on your program is the fuel you can use to feed your motivational engine. It's important to recognize success as it comes and not always have your sights on the ultimate goal. For example, I was working with someone, PR, who wanted to lose 50 pounds in six months. This was an ambitious but realistic goal. We had decided to make mini goals so that she could focus not on the big number that seemed so far away but on smaller numbers that were attainable and that would keep her encouraged as she plotted her course to the finish line. One day she proudly e-mailed me that she had made progress. I thought she was going to report that she had exceeded her weekly weight-loss goal. Instead, she wrote that she had gone to the movies on Saturday and did something she hadn't done in years: She sat through the movie without eating one kernel of popcorn. She admitted to missing it but was proud that she could munch away on her bag of baby carrots and leave the theater knowing she had been disciplined and hadn't jeopardized all the hard work and great results she had seen up to that point.

Success begets success. This can be one of your biggest motivators to continue doing what you're doing and see the journey to the end.

MOTIVATIONAL EXERCISE

Another way to find your motivational engine is to create a motivation table. List at least five things you want to do or are supposed to do on your weight-loss program and then for each item list the advantages and disadvantages. Below is what a table might look like.

THINGS YOU WANT TO DO (THE ACTION)	BENEFITS	DISADVANTAGES
Eat more fruits and vegetables.	Healthier food. More vitamins and nutrients. Lower calories. Better for weight loss. Contain antioxidants.	Don't like the taste.
Exercise regularly.	Burn calories. Lose weight faster. Improve overall health. Live longer.	I'm lazy. This makes me move. I have to find the time in my busy day. I don't like messing up my hair.
Drink only 1 soda a day.	Save calories for healthier food. Reduce unnecessary sugars. Increase water consumption.	Miss the energy boost from the caffeine. Miss the taste. Other drinks don't taste as good with my food.
Don't eat within 90 minutes of sleeping.	Calories don't sit around and get converted to fat while I'm sleeping. Better chance to burn off the food calories. Better for digestion.	Have to plan my meals better. Busy schedule makes this difficult to do every night. Might get hungry before I go to bed.
Cut down on fried foods.	Fewer calories. Better for my cholesterol levels. Better for my heart and blood vessels. Makes losing weight easier.	Miss the flavor. Easy to find. Less expensive.

Once you have completed your chart, it's time to understand what your answers mean. Compare what's listed in the advantages column to what's listed in the disadvantages column. If the advantages column not only makes sense but is feasible, then you're off to a good start at finding motivation. The next thing you need to do is ask which of the columns seems to be more impactful in your life. Do the benefits in your mind outweigh the discomfort, inconvenience, and other negatives of the disadvantages? For example, does cutting down on fried foods and improving cholesterol levels and your heart and blood vessel health and losing weight feel more important than missing the flavor, taking more time to find healthier food, and possibly spending a little more money for those items that will deliver greater benefit? If the answer is yes, then you've tapped into something. This comparison is what you must remind yourself of when you decide to do what's "right."

What if you feel that the disadvantages column is stronger than the benefits column? This is a problem that you need to analyze and hopefully resolve. One strategy I like is the compromise. Maybe there are some boxes where you're willing to endure the disadvantages for the benefits of the action. See how many boxes they add up to. For the sake of our example, let's say boxes 1, 4, and 5 are fine, and you're willing to commit to the action for the sake of the benefit even though there are disadvantages. What to do with boxes 2 and 3?

When you find yourself conflicted over certain boxes, the best thing to do is take your time to work it out mentally first, before jumping right in and doing the action. What you don't want is to have such an unpleasant experience that you will forever swear off doing the behavior again. If possible, try to take the action in stages. For example, perhaps you're studying the conflicted box 3—reducing your soda consumption to one a day. Let's say you absolutely enjoy drinking soda, and you typically consume four cans a day. One way of working toward resolving the conflict might consist of reducing your consumption not to one a day but three a day. Then every two weeks cut back one more until you eventually reach one a day as your program suggests. This phased approach is a way to keep motivated without feeling overwhelmed.

S.M.A.R.T.E.R. FOOD CHOICES: THE GLYCEMIC INDEX AT WORK

You've probably heard of the glycemic index. Nutritionists and diet experts alike have embraced this classification of foods because it can be a powerful guide to making smarter food choices. Rather than bore you with the scientific details of how the index works, let me cut to the chase. The glycemic index ranks foods based on how fast the body breaks them down into simple sugar, which you might also know as glucose. It stands to reason that the faster a food is broken down into sugar, the faster and higher the levels of sugar rise in the blood. The faster your blood sugar levels rise, the stronger the

Work Box

MOTIVATIONAL SOURCE QUESTIONS

1. Name three things you've accomplished in life that have made you proud.

2. In the past when you've tried to accomplish something difficult and the odds were stacked against you, what inspired you to continue and eventually succeed?

3. If you faced a physical challenge sometime in your life (finishing a race while exhausted; carrying bags of groceries when your hands and arms were begging you to put the groceries down; walking a long distance under tough weather conditions but not giving up) or have gone the extra distance such as studying for long hours to pass a test or finish a work assignment, what did you mentally focus on to get you through the pain, the discomfort, and the temptation to quit?

4. Is there someone in your life you would do almost anything for?

CREATE FIVE AFFIRMATIONS

_____

_____

_____

_____

_____

(continued)

COMPLETE YOUR MOTIVATION TABLE

THINGS YOU WANT TO DO	BENEFITS	DISADVANTAGES

signal that is sent to your pancreas (a small fish-shaped organ that sits behind the stomach and makes hormones such as insulin and enzymes that help the body digest food) to release the insulin hormone into the blood.

Insulin is an extremely important hormone because it sweeps up excess sugar from the blood and brings it into the cells where it can be used right away as a source of energy, stored for future use in the form of glycogen, or stored as the dreaded fat if the body doesn't need energy at that particular time. As you can imagine, it's this last process that haunts anyone trying to lose weight. The higher the glycemic index, the faster the food is broken down into sugar, the more insulin gets released, the more sugar is swept into the cells, and the more fat gets packed onto the body. You want to eat a diet that is not only lower in calories but *also* low on the glycemic index.

High GI	Medium GI	Low GI
>70	56–69	<55

LOW GI FOODS			
FOOD	GLYCEMIC INDEX (GLUCOSE=100)	SERVING SIZE	CARBOHYDRATES PER SERVING (G)
Dates, dried	103	2 oz	40
Corn flakes	81	1 cup	26
Jelly beans	78	1 oz	28
Puffed rice cakes	78	3 cakes	21
Russet potato (baked)	76	1 large	30
Doughnut	76	1 large	23
Soda crackers	74	4 crackers	17
White bread	73	1 large slice	14
Table sugar (sucrose)	68	2 tsp	10
Pancake	67	6" diameter	58
White rice (boiled)	64	1 cup	36
Brown rice (boiled)	55	1 cup	33
Spaghetti, white (boiled 10–15 min)	44	1 cup	40
Orange	42	1 large	11
Rye or pumpernickel bread	41	1 large slice	12
Spaghetti, white (boiled 5 min)	38	1 cup	40
Pear	38	1 large	11
Apple	38	1 large	15
All-Bran cereal	38	1 cup	23

(continued)

LOW GI FOODS			
FOOD	GLYCEMIC INDEX (GLUCOSE=100)	SERVING SIZE	CARBOHYDRATES PER SERVING (G)
Spaghetti, whole wheat (boiled)	37	1 cup	37
Skim milk	32	8 oz	13
Lentils, dried (boiled)	29	1 cup	18
Kidney beans, dried (boiled)	28	1 cup	25
Pearl barley (boiled)	25	1 cup	42
Cashew nuts	22	1 oz	9
Peanuts	14	1 oz	6

Source: K. Foster-Powell, S. H. Holt, and J. C. Brand-Miller, "International Table of Glycemic Index and Glycemic Load Values: 2002," American Journal of Clinical Nutrition 76, no. 1 (2002): 5–56.

CHAPTER 4

Resist Temptation

YOUR MIND MUST LEAD YOU

Is it easy resisting temptation? Absolutely not, but this chapter will help you stay resolved in the face of it. Let's establish context first. Temptations are abundantly and conveniently located throughout our environment. Whether it's that expensive designer scarf that you want so badly but know it's beyond your budget, eavesdropping on a conversation between an arguing couple at the table next to yours, or a piece of double fudge chocolate cake—the temptations are endless. The good news is that we are successful more times than not at resisting the urges to indulge in these forbidden callings. So why do we lose on occasion and give in to temptation? What happens late at night when you can't stop yourself from downing a handful of chocolate chip cookies or plucking off the lid to that pint of butter pecan ice cream? It's about the mind losing its competitive edge.

One way of thinking about temptation is as a fierce conflict, one that you can win if you focus mentally and train properly. When it comes to resisting temptation, your mind is locked in an epic battle with your anticipated sense of physical satisfaction. Your body knows that buying that scarf, eavesdropping on the juicy details of that argument, or biting into that double fudge cake will produce a physical response of pleasure. Your challenge is to convince yourself that the brief reward you get from the indulgence will be less pleasurable than the reward you get from abstaining. In other words, you have to train your mind, strengthen it, and prepare it to recognize and seek the more enduring pleasure—a pleasure that does not provide immediate gratification but can be extremely satisfying over the long term.

Before we begin to train your brain, you must first be convinced that you *can* resist all those temptations lurking in vending machines, bakeries, and fast-food restaurants. If you believe that it's possible to develop the mental willpower to succeed, then this increases your chances dramatically. Any doubt or skepticism will only reduce your chances of ultimate success. Keep telling yourself that your mind is strong enough to keep your body under control. The discipline you learn and exhibit in this phase of your program can prove useful not only in your weight-loss efforts but on the larger stage of life.

TRAIN YOUR BRAIN

UNDERSTANDING THE PHYSICAL

Why do we eat foods even when we know they will keep us from losing weight? Getting to that answer means understanding pleasure and the body's physical response to it. Scientists have believed for years that the neurotransmitter dopamine, a chemical found in the brain, is the brain's "pleasure chemical," sending signals between brain cells in a way to reward a person for a particular activity. The precise details of this pleasure loop haven't been completely determined, but enough of it has been clarified to give us an idea of why the body commits us to actions that are against what we know makes sense for that body.

The neurons—nerve cells in the brain—that produce dopamine seem to activate just *before* the pleasurable activity is engaged. The timing of what comes first is still being worked out, but one leading theory is that our brain releases a certain amount of dopamine in anticipation of how pleasurable we expect the activity is going to be. The dopamine then becomes a motivator as it increases our energy and drive to participate in the pleasurable activity. The more pleasurable the activity, the higher the dopamine levels, the more vigorously we pursue and engage in the activity. If you don't find the activity as pleasurable as you expected, your dopamine levels decrease and you lose interest.

The brain's dopamine reward system can be extremely strong depending on the degree of pleasure one achieves. For example, take warm apple pie and vanilla ice cream. For many people, eating this dessert produces such a level of pleasure and satisfaction that they find it almost impossible to pass up the opportunity to order it when seeing it on a restaurant menu or being served to another diner. The dopamine response to the thought, sight, smell, and taste of the apple pie is overpowering, and despite great efforts to avoid the sugary dessert, they simply can't help themselves.

CRAVINGS

We've all had a craving—a strong desire to eat or drink something, so strong we can't get the thought of it out of our minds. Most people think of cravings as intense urges that gnaw at the body and mind until the desired item is consumed. But scientists aren't so sure where cravings come from or why they exist. One long-held belief is that when we are calorie starved or deficient of certain nutrients, we crave what we're missing, whether it's carbohydrates, fat, or protein. The craving serves as the body's alarm clock to let it know that the level of that particular type of fuel is getting dangerously low and it's time to do something about it—eat.

Another popular theory is that when we eat the right combination of fat and carbohydrates that have pleasurable tastes and textures, our body builds up a memory of satisfaction and seeks to repeat it in the future. In essence, the body craves those foods that make it feel good. Some leading nutritionists have even drawn the conclusion that cravings are connected to hormones. That theory says that as we age we become less hormonal and the frequency of our cravings diminishes drastically.

80–20 RULE

No one is perfect, and no one is going to follow any particular diet program perfectly. In fact, it's advantageous at times to indulge in some of the "fun" foods that your program might consider off limits. Some diets go too far in eliminating too many foods. If something is completely prohibited, it's too easy to focus on it. One of the dangers this imposes is that you become obsessed with those "off-limit" foods, which increases the temptation and pressure to eat them. It's fine to have a "cheat" every once in a while; in fact, some programs even call for a cheat day. The truth of the matter is that eating an extra cookie or scoop of ice cream occasionally is not going to sabotage your program. That's why I believe in the 80–20 rule. If 80 percent of what you eat is healthy and on the program and the remaining 20 percent is off the program, you will still be successful at losing weight.

The reason many programs don't want to allow for cheating, however, is that most people don't know when to stop. One cheat can lead to a bigger cheat that leads to an even bigger cheat, and then you're off the program. You have to be the judge of your discipline level. If you're someone who gets a taste of chocolate or french fries and can't stop yourself from eating the entire package or serving, then this method is not for you. You'd be better off following the program as closely as possible with a goal of staying away from those temptations that tend to lead you to overeat.

IDENTIFY YOUR TRIGGERS

Most of the tempting foods you crave tend to be "forbidden" on a weight-loss program. High-calorie items such as french fries, sugar-frosted pastries, and chocolate can invade your thoughts and suddenly appear to overpower your physical ability to ignore the craving.

To get a better grasp of how to deal with your temptations or cravings, it's important to identify what triggers you to indulge. The simple exercise that follows will give you a clearer understanding of which environmental/emotional/physical stimuli have you reaching for forbidden foods. See the sample chart on the facing page. List your cravings/temptations in the column on the left-hand side of a piece of paper and then list the stimulus that drives you to eat each item in the column on the right side of the paper.

Identifying your triggers is an important first step; now it's time to do something about them. Take each temptation and try to find an alternate way to deal with the emotion that leads to your indulgence. For example, if you tend to reach for ice cream after you've had an argument or when you're upset, then it's time to figure out other ways to channel your anger. Exercise is not only a great way to blow off some steam, but you can expend your nervous

TEMPTING FOODS	TRIGGER
Buttered popcorn	Watching TV
Cherry licorice	Boredom
Chocolate	Nervous / anxious
Cookies	After-work hunger
Creamy pasta	Stressed
Doughnuts/pastries	In a rush and hungry
French fries	In the car driving home
Ice cream	Arguments/anger
Pizza	Too tired to cook, ordering in
Soda	When I need energy

energy in a way that will help you lose weight. Taking a 15-minute walk out-side and enjoying nature is another way to settle down and slow your racing heartbeat. There are numerous other physical and mental activities—from deep yoga-style breathing to walking the dog—that can come to soothe you much more than a forbidden food fest ever could.

Sometimes visual instead of emotional triggers can be the problem. Someone once told me how she craved french fries. She simply couldn't stop herself from eating them regardless of how often she told herself the fries were ruining her weight-loss efforts. I asked her a few questions and discovered that she only got the cravings driving home from work. The route she drove took her down a street that had both Burger King and McDonald's within a couple of hundred yards of each other. Some days she could make it past McDonald's, only to turn into the Burger King lot a couple of minutes later. Other days she couldn't get past McDonald's. The fix for this was easy: Don't drive past the restaurants. By adjusting her route so that she got off the expressway one exit early and drove a different set of streets to get home, she added only five minutes to her drive but eliminated her usual trigger, making it to her house without the craving for fries. If your cravings are attached to visual stimuli, figure out a way to avoid seeing that stimulus. It's always a great strategy to replace unhealthy routines with healthy ones.

VISUALIZE THE CONSEQUENCE

The key to overcoming temptation is to strengthen your mind so that triggers no longer overpower your resistance. One method I've found helpful is to teach your mind how to visualize the consequence of your action. Let's say you're craving a bowl of creamy fettuccine Alfredo. Satisfying that craving could be as simple as picking up the phone and ordering delivery from your favorite restaurant. Within the hour you could be happily finishing off the bowl of tasty pasta. Then what? You've satisfied the craving, but now you've dumped almost 900 whopping calories into your body. Visualize the consequences. You'd have to run almost 7 miles, ride a stationary bicycle for two hours, or hit a punching bag for two hours to burn off the equivalent of what you just consumed in one bowl of pasta. Imagine all the fat inside that creamy sauce pouring into your arteries, narrowing the opening through which your blood is trying to flow. The more of that creamy sauce you eat, the narrower the opening becomes and the greater the chance of your suffering a heart attack or stroke. Imagine yourself in a dressing room barely squeezing into a pair of pants and not being able to button them because all that creamy pasta is building up a fortress of fat around your midsection.

Is the *temporary* satisfaction you got from eating that pasta worth the consequences? This is the type of pro-con question you must always ask yourself when faced with temptation. You should also consider the context. The pasta gratification may be immediate and thrilling, but it is short term and will quickly fade. The long-term gratification of not eating the pasta and sticking to your plan of losing weight can be a more satisfying thrill, especially when you move closer to your goal, start wearing clothes that you haven't been able to fit into in years, or your doctor takes you off medications for your high blood pressure, diabetes, or high cholesterol. Each situation should lead you to a quick cost-benefit analysis, and if you do the correct calculations, you'll find that the long-term cost of indulging in your craving far outweighs the short-term benefit.

KEEP OUT OF REACH

If it's not there, you can't eat it. This seems like a simple strategy that shouldn't need repeating, but it's one that too many people don't use. Why stock your cabinets and freezers with foods that you know you're either not supposed to eat or you're supposed to consume in small amounts? You are tempting yourself unnecessarily and creating a conflict between your mind and your body.

Controlling your food environment is a smart way to avoid making yourself vulnerable to temptation. Your home environment isn't the only thing you'd be smart to regulate. The workplace can be an equally dangerous place. Don't keep jars of candy and finger foods stocked in or on your desk. Vending machines are another "hot" area to be avoided at all cost. Avoid the cafeteria or the hallway where these "temptation depots" are ominously lurking, waiting to draw you into their *sugartopia*.

Don't forget about all those office parties and social events that will be full of tasty but fattening food. You will undoubtedly be offered limitless alcohol, but don't be fooled. Alcohol is nothing more than liquid calories. Many mistakenly believe that because alcohol is liquid it's not as bad as eating a cheeseburger and fries. A calorie is a calorie. Whether it's from liquid alcohol or fried foods, the calorie will still add pounds on the scale and cholesterol in your arteries.

CREATE A TEMPTATION PLAN

Temptations won't suddenly disappear from your environment. Since temptation is a permanent part of the world we live in, it's best to create a plan to deal with it. This plan must be portable, easily accessible, and simple enough to be activated at a moment's notice. My high school basketball coach would call it the lesson of the five P's: *Proper Preparation Prevents Poor Performance.* If you prepare for the possibility of temptation, then you'll perform well when it's time to resist whatever is trying to reel you in.

Forming a plan is as easy as adding more information to your trigger chart. Pull out the chart and make a third column that lists a response you can choose instead of giving in to the tempting food. Your modified chart might look something like this:

Copy your chart on an index card and keep it with you at all times. When you have new ideas for ways to distract yourself from temptation, add them to the chart. Make several copies and keep them strategically placed so that whether

TEMPTING FOODS	TRIGGER	ALTERNATIVE BEHAVIOR
Chocolate	Nervous/anxious	Call your support buddy and discuss.
Buttered popcorn	Watching TV	Snack on raw, crunchy veggies.
Ice cream	Arguments/anger	Exercise; write in your journal.
Cookies	After-work hunger	Grab a 100-calorie snack pack.
French fries	In the car driving home	Change your route home.
Pizza	Too tired to cook, ordering in	Rotate delivery menus.
Doughnuts/pastries	In a rush and hungry	Keep fresh fruit handy.
Cherry licorice	Boredom	Get active; pursue a hobby; brush your teeth.
Creamy pasta	Stressed	Listen to relaxation music/meditate.
Soda	When I need energy	Try unsweetened caffeinated tea.

you're at home, work, or running errands, you can quickly reach a copy and activate your plan.

GO AHEAD AND ENJOY—WITHIN REASON

There is enough convincing evidence that avoiding cravings might only make the cravings stronger and more frequent. In fact, some nutritional psychologists urge their patients to listen to their cravings and respond accordingly by eating a small amount of what they crave. Moderation is, of course, the part that can be tricky. Many people who get a taste of that tempting food can't stop themselves from overeating. But there are a couple of ways that you can help satisfy your taste for something sweet or chocolaty and not overdo it on the calories.

Portion out your cheats in advance (or have someone else do it for you if handling the indulgent food is too tempting for you at this point). To avoid eating too much, divide any food into smaller allotments. For example, let's say you have a craving for Oreo cookie ice cream. When you purchase the ice cream, don't store it in your freezer in the original packaging. Instead, purchase smaller disposable containers. Gladware and other brands make some great disposable snack-size bowls with lids. Take the pint or quart of ice cream and divide it into small one-scoop portions and store them in the individual containers. Stack the one-scoop containers in the freezer. Now when you have an urge, you can go ahead and have the ice cream, but allow yourself only one container at a time, which means one scoop. Whether it's putting chips into a smaller Ziploc bag or slicing up that candy bar and refrigerating it in sections, you can plan ahead to satisfy those cravings without overindulging.

BALANCE YOUR PLATE

Our bodies will often crave what we're missing in our meal plan. Programs that call for severely restricting the variety of foods you eat can inadvertently create a deficit and thus goad you to eat those missing foods. If possible, keep as much diversity in your meal as possible. Try to eat some carbohydrates, fat, and protein at as many meals as possible. Remember that protein and fat take longer to digest, so you'll feel full longer and decrease the likelihood of cravings. Or use the dinner plate trick: Mentally bisect your plate and load half of it with vegetables and fruits. Then bisect the remaining half and divide protein, fats, and carbohydrates between the sections.

Fiber can be another important weapon in your struggle against temptation. Fiber is a special type of carbohydrate that is found mostly in the outer layers of plants. Unlike the other food substances we consume, fiber passes through the body's digestive system without being broken down into smaller nutrients. Adult women should shoot for a daily consumption of 20 grams or more of fiber; men should shoot for 30 grams or more. The average American eats less than half of these recommended amounts. The benefits of fiber are extensive and include the following:

Requires us to chew more and thus slows down the eating process, increasing our feeling of fullness without adding calories.

Slows digestion and absorption so that the sugar in food enters the blood more slowly, thus keeping blood sugar levels even, rather than causing spikes and lows.

Makes food more satisfying by increasing the bulk of the stomach contents and staying there longer before moving down the digestive tract.

Fiber has also been cited as helping to lower blood-cholesterol levels and to reduce rates of colon cancer and heart and kidney disease. See the chart below for some great sources of fiber.

KEEP BUSY

I have talked to many people who have struggled with resisting cravings and asked them for their secrets. One of the most common answers I got was the success of distraction. When they felt the urge or a craving, they would simply distract themselves with either a physical or a mental activity. One person told me that every time she got the urge to eat a Drake's Devil Dog, she would go outside and work in her garden, and after twenty minutes she'd be so engaged with her work that the urge to have the crème-filled snack would pass. Others

Common Dietary Sources of Fiber

- Apples
- Barley
- Beans
- Blueberries
- Brown rice
- Bulgur
- Carrots
- Celery
- Couscous
- Cucumbers
- Dried peas

- Legumes (beans)
- Lentils
- Nuts and seeds
- Oatmeal, oat bran
- Pears
- Strawberries
- Tomatoes
- Wheat bran
- Whole wheat bread
- Whole-grain breakfast cereals
- Zucchini

Source: Harvard School of Public Health

Work Box

1. Identify your food triggers.

2. Visualize and then list the consequences of giving in to your temptation.

3. Create your temptation plan.

would grab the newspaper and begin working on a crossword puzzle. Someone else told me he just picked up the phone and called his girlfriend. The idea is simple. Keeping your mind and hands otherwise engaged leaves little time for you to think about or give in to that temptation.

CHAPTER 5

Think Thin

YOU ARE WHAT YOU THINK YOU ARE

The mind-body connection is something that ancient philosophers discussed, even though their contemporaries widely criticized them. The power of thought—more specifically, what I like to call *directional thought*—is difficult to study by Western scientific methods. But just because a concept doesn't fit neatly into Western science's "acceptable" studies doesn't mean that it doesn't have validity. If nothing else, the idea of "mind over body" is certainly nothing new.

For years many sports psychologists have written about the mind's ability to control the body. If you want to be a winner, you have to think like a winner. If you want to be successful at losing weight, you have to think like someone who has successfully *lost* weight. The mind has the uncanny ability to power the body and take it beyond its perceived physical limits. I can remember my childhood baseball and basketball coaches stressing how important it was to "think positive." I particularly remember my high school basketball coach, Dan Murphy, with his wide eyes and eternally hoarse voice. One of our daily exercises during practice was shooting free throws. According to Coach Murphy, most games were won or lost based on a team's ability to sink those free throws, especially during the critical last few minutes of a game. Every week we spent hours doing drills that required our sinking a certain number of conservative free throws in order to move on to the next drill in practice.

One day our big man, Bryan Patzer, was on the line; he needed to make two shots in a row for the practice to end. Every time he missed one of the two, the entire team had to run a wind sprint and then line up again as Patzer attempted to make two consecutive shots. Well, Patzer was normally a reliable free throw shooter, but he was a big guy and it was the end of practice and we were all exhausted. His legs and arms were weak, which meant his technique and shooting rhythm were badly out of sync. Patzer would make the first shot and then miss the second shot or miss the first shot, which sent us running again. This pattern was repeated over and over for about fifteen minutes. After about five sprints, our tongues were mopping up the floor. Coach Murphy walked over from the sideline and grabbed the ball out of Patzer's hands. He got within an inch of Patzer's face, his eyes bulging, and screamed: "Dammit, Patzer. You have to *will* the ball into the basket!" Patzer looked at him as if he wanted to punch his lights out, but Coach Murphy didn't let up. "When you're tired and your body is giving out and you need to make the shot, your mind has to take over for your body and *will* that ball into the basket."

After two hours of a grueling practice with my legs feeling like rubber, I was with Patzer—I thought Coach Murphy was just riding the big man and off on one of his philosophical rants, which he was prone to do. But as the season wore on and we came to critical points in competitive games where we needed to make those free throws, Coach Murphy would get up from his seat on the sidelines, look at us with that look, and mouth the words, "*Will* it into the basket." To our surprise, this worked more often than not and helped us win a lot games.

Why did it work? I've spent a lot of time thinking about that over the years. I started to use Coach Murphy's mental technique in my own life. When trying to accomplish something difficult, I would think back to those basketball practices and hear Coach Murphy's voice fill the gymnasium. I inevitably felt more empowered to complete the task. What we hadn't realized in basketball practice was that Coach Murphy hadn't just been teaching us how to make free throws; he had been teaching us the power of the mind and how important it was to let our mental focus power the physical. I've used Coach Murphy's mantra when trying to finish a tough workout in the gym or staying up late into the night to work through a long list of must-finish assignments. You can use the same mental technique on your weight-loss journey.

If you think you are overweight or unhealthy or a failure, then you are going to be just that. But if you *will* yourself to be thin or healthy or successful, then that is the direction you will move in and ultimately achieve your goal. Of course, just thinking you are thin is not all it takes to lose weight or maintain weight loss, but positive thinking can power your body to stay on track and make thinking about success a self-fulfilling prophecy. Our minds can be like the strings that control the limbs of a puppet. Cut those strings, and the puppeteer no longer has control over the puppet's movement. Lose your mental focus, and eventually you will stall on your program or, even worse, gain weight.

UNLOCK YOURSELF FROM THE PRISON OF FAT

I have worked directly and indirectly with thousands of people who have struggled to lose weight. They have tried multiple programs, spent large sums of money, and quit those programs over and over. I worked with one famous singer who, while she wasn't happy with her weight, had grown comfortable with it. Her record company and manager disagreed, however, and insisted that she lose weight. She was told in no uncertain terms that success in the music business was not just about a singer's voice or catchy lyrics but also about the company's ability to market the artist as a package, which of course includes how one looks. In that industry's ultracompetitive environment, a singer's appearance was just as important as how well she could hit her notes.

The singer started her weight-loss plan and was determined to succeed. She had a couple of food weaknesses that we had to work around, but for the most part she changed her diet and increased her exercise. Her results were immediate and steady. Every week she was down 2 or 3 pounds. I was pleased with her results on the scale and also was encouraged that she was making lifestyle changes that would not just get her looking great for her album cover but help her be healthy the rest of her life.

Seven weeks into the program she weighed in and was down 16 pounds. Her goal was 25 pounds, which meant she was well within striking distance. I couldn't be happier about her progress, but when I revealed how much she had lost, I was surprised by her reaction. Disappointment was written across her face.

"What's wrong?" I asked. "You're down sixteen pounds, nine away from your goal. You're doing great."

"I don't feel great," she said. "I'm still fat. I don't see any progress."

"What do you mean?" I asked. "You're down sixteen pounds. It's evident in your face and midsection. The scale isn't lying."

"I know the scale says what it says, and I believe it, but I still feel fat," the singer said, her voice breaking. "I look in the mirror, and I can't see a difference."

Was she just saying these things because she wanted me to compliment her and say how well she was doing? Compliment-seeking is not uncommon for people losing weight, nor is it necessarily a bad thing. People who work hard to achieve—especially in an area where they've failed before—like and need to hear some praise about their efforts. Positive reinforcement is a good thing.

But then the singer started crying. That's when I knew it wasn't an act, and this was not about seeking compliments.

"You're down two dress sizes, your face is thinner, and clothes that were tight on you a couple of months ago are too big," I said. "How can you not feel thinner?"

"I don't know," she shrugged. "I just don't see the difference."

"What do your friends say?"

"That I look a lot smaller. They can see I've lost weight."

"But you don't?"

She shook her head.

That's when it dawned on me: She knew by all objective measures (scale and clothes) that she had lost weight, but her mind wouldn't accept her new body. Her eyes saw a slimmer body, but her mind blocked that image from imprinting on her brain. She couldn't process it. In essence, the singer was a prisoner trapped in her own perception of fat. I realized that my work with her needed to extend beyond administering and supervising her diet plan. I had to diagnose and help remedy whatever was going on above her shoulders. Like thousands of others who had lost weight but couldn't see it, she was unable to shed that image of being overweight, an image that she had accepted for so long. This image hadn't prevented her from sticking to the plan and losing weight, but there was a tremendous risk that if she continued to see herself as failing, she might ignore the very real progress she was making on the scale and quit the program. When losing weight, the mind needs to be nourished as much as the body.

How does one start accepting and celebrating success? One exercise that can be extremely helpful is focusing on the positives. People who have lost weight but still see themselves as overweight can typically find at least a few things about their bodies that they like. It could be their hair, fingernails, eyes, or some other body part. Stand in front of a mirror to canvas the things that you find appealing and focus on them. If you don't like the width of your hips or size of your thighs, then don't pay attention to them. Enjoy all the parts you do find attractive and over time start incorporating those less appealing areas into the "appealing group" until you accept your entire body as something worthy of pride rather than shame.

Do things that confirm and affirm you have lost weight. Go to the store and have fun trying on and buying new clothes that are a smaller size and accentuate your new physique. One dieter I worked with for over a year said that her greatest moment of triumph in a long time had been going to one of her favorite stores and being sent away from the plus-size department to one of the floors that carried smaller sizes. Before that shopping trip, I had been telling her how great she looked, as had many of her colleagues and her friends. But it wasn't until the salesclerk explained that she could no longer fit their plus sizes that she accepted and celebrated her new body.

ACT THIN

A business partner and I recently had a meeting in Chicago with a well-respected journalist. I had known the journalist for many years, but this was the first time my partner was meeting him. When she and I were waiting for him to enter the conference room, I explained to her that he had lost over 200 pounds in the last few years and was a different person not just physically but also in his perspective on life, health, and priorities.

A few minutes later RM entered the room. I remembered him 200 plus pounds ago, so seeing him much slimmer and energized brought an immediate smile to my face. The introductions were made, we had a great meeting, and then my partner and I left the building and were walking to our car. "So what do you think?" I asked her.

"It went really well," she said. Then she stopped walking. "But there was something strange about him that kept nagging at me."

"What's that?" I asked.

"You said he lost over two hundred pounds, right?"

I nodded.

"But does he know that he lost two hundred pounds?"

"Of course he does." I laughed. "That's a ridiculous question. It's his body."

"Well, he sure doesn't act as if he's lost all that weight," she said.

"What do you mean?"

"He still acts big," she said.

We stopped walking again.

"How?"

"He's wearing a suit that's several sizes too big, and he still walks like a big person."

When she said this, I felt that a thunderbolt had just struck my brain. Her observations explained the mental disconnect that occurs when the mind of someone who has lost weight hasn't caught up. Then I thought of RM. His coat was so big that the shoulders were falling to his chest. His pants were so loose around the waist that wide gaps of cloth were bunched up and held together by his belt. And he had that "big man walk," the one where the legs are spread wide, and instead of walking, it's more like plodding—one foot following the other in a very labored and methodical manner. His body and mind were not synchronized.

Why do people who have lost weight still dress and carry themselves like their former big selves? I spoke with several people who found themselves in this predicament as well as psychologists who have treated people with a similar mind-body disconnect. What I learned was eye-opening. It's not uncommon for people to find it difficult to accept their physical transformation, and many of these people harbor a fear of their own success. This was exactly the opposite of what I expected. Logic says if someone has worked diligently to lose weight and has made sacrifices and lifestyle changes, they would enthusiastically embrace the fruits of their labor. When a sporting team wins a championship, they don't stand up in front of their screaming fans and television cameras and review all the reasons why they don't deserve the trophy. They celebrate their victory and the hard work that went into winning the prize.

When someone has been overweight for a long time, it's difficult to accept a new reality, even if the reality is something they've dreamed of attaining and have worked tirelessly to attain. To avoid this, you need to make mental adjustments just as your body is adapting to its new weight and shape. This means that you need to start *acting thin* the second you lose your first pound. I'm not saying you should throw on a bikini and parade up and down the beach on day one. But what I'm saying is make an effort to break those "big person habits." Stop sitting in the front of the bus because you don't want people to watch you walking to a seat toward the back. Stop sitting in the back of the theater to avoid having people watch you walk down the aisle. Stop wearing baggy pants and bulky sweaters to hide the bulges.

Your new body most likely means you have greater physical endurance then you are used to. Don't be afraid to use the stairs along with others instead of the elevator. You can probably walk greater distances now, so don't waste time trying to park your car in the spot nearest the entrance. When you start acting thin and thinking thin, you pull yourself clear of outdated thinking about your size, and this means your mind will be ready to take on new challenges and enjoy all the progress you've worked so hard to achieve.

DON'T FEAR SUCCESS

I had never met a person who feared success until I started working with a highly successful corporate executive who was on a mission to lose weight and take back control of her life. PR had been dieting for most of her adult life, fluctuating by as much as 20 pounds depending on the time of year and her level of dedication. We had been working together on and off for almost fourteen months, and she had turned the corner these last two months. She was the most serious she had been since we started, setting a new and ambitious goal and tapping into her motivational engines. She wanted this success, and she wanted it badly.

She had just completed two extremely successful months of continuous weight loss and lifestyle changes that had her making better decisions about her diet and exercise. Once a week she weighed herself and reported the number to me. According to my notes, she was on the verge of reaching a significant milestone in her journey. She was about to lose 40 pounds and hit a number that she hadn't weighed in more than ten years.

One night I was on a trip and received a Blackberry message from her that she needed to speak to me right away and to please call her when my plane landed. The message was so brief and direct, it made me think something terrible had happened. I called her as soon as we hit the tarmac. She answered in a low voice. I asked her what was wrong, and she told me: She had just weighed herself and hit the lowest number she could remember in over a decade. I could hear the tears in her voice.

We talked more, congratulating and thanking each other, and then planning how she was going to reach her 50-pound weight-loss milestone. We were in uncharted territory, so it was important to think through the next steps carefully. The next day I e-mailed her a four-day plan. This plan was no different in difficulty or intensity from the previous plans I had made for her, but the stakes were even higher. She had an extremely important presentation to make in a week and she wanted to look her best.

She completed the first day and, as was our custom, e-mailed me her daily eating/exercise journal at the end of the day. I was smiling as I read through the details of her consumption and physical activity log. She had followed my program to the letter. Then I got to the "comments" section of her message, and my smile quickly evaporated. This is what she wrote:

> For some reason this suddenly feels HARD! I don't know what has happened, but I'm having difficulty with the plan. I don't know what it is.

The day she had just completed was by no means one of the more difficult days. She had successfully completed much more rigorous parts of the program that required strict nutritional discipline and intense exercise. But for the first time in three months she was complaining about the program. Was it a coincidence that her complaint was registered only one day after she hit the biggest milestone of her journey?

I thought about it for a while and then pieced it all together. The timing was not a coincidence. She felt this had been a "hard" day not because it was too intense or had asked too much of her, but because she was afraid. She had come face-to-face with success, and now she had to make a decision. She could continue to do the right things she had been doing for the last several months and reach even greater heights, or she could start slipping, return to her previous poor decision-making and behaviors, and start gaining weight. As far as choices go, this sounded like a no-brainer, but when I took a deeper look, it was a lot more complicated than it first appeared. This is the rest of our e-mail exchange:

I wrote:

> You are at the CRITICAL moment of success. Don't let anything or anyone turn you back. This is all about YOU! You've worked too hard and come too far to let it slip away. Others would kill to be where you are right now, standing at the crossroads of opportunity to change your life forever. Don't run away from it. Take it head-on like a champ!!!

She wrote:

> I just reread what you wrote. You said something critical that I think I have done in my past unsuccessful weight-loss efforts. You said don't run away from it. I think in the past, I get close and then turn around and run away. I don't know why and no one has ever used those words to challenge me. You struck a cord that I didn't even know was there. It's heavy on my mind and will help me get thru the next 3 days.

The next day I received this message:

> I really think I am resisting the success. It's not like me in most areas of my life, but my weight is different. I am going to plow through this awkward period. The visualization helps. The deadline of next Monday on that stage is the driver.

My client was an extremely intelligent, fiercely competitive, highly accomplished corporate executive who was afraid of winning what was arguably the biggest battle of her life. She had not only expressed in no uncertain terms that she wanted the success, but she had gone to great lengths to make sure she attained it. Yet after drawing closer to the ultimate goal than she ever had before, her mind and body started rejecting the possibility of success. Why?

Some fear successful weight loss because they're actually afraid that this new physical transformation will make them more attractive. In their mind, this new attractiveness could change a lot of things in their life that have been stable (and comforting) for a long time. They start wondering if others will now look at a thinner person and automatically view what they do and say from a negative perspective. ("She's only saying that because she's lost weight and thinks she's hot stuff." "Ever since she lost that weight and got a new wardrobe she's been all attitude.") The possibility that others might misinterpret or incorrectly attribute blame to weight-loss success is enough to make some people nervous and even fearful of putting themselves in that position.

I worked with a famous comedian who had said he wanted to lose weight but not *too* much weight. I told him that I thought he should lose only enough to give him a healthy BMI. Even after I explained to him the significant health and appearance benefits of his potential new weight, he still didn't want to lose the bulk of his heft. At first I couldn't understand why he was being so resistant, but the ensuing conversation explained it all.

DR. IAN: You've already lost almost half of your goal and, you're looking great. Why don't you want to lose the rest of it? You'll feel better and look better.

JL: But then I won't be funny.

DR. IAN: What are you talking about? Of course you'll still be funny. Losing weight won't affect your ability to tell a good joke.

JL: But you don't understand. People like me and feel comfortable around me because I'm the fat guy. I'm funny because I'm the fat guy, and people think it's okay to laugh with me. If I lose too much weight, I'll be the thin guy trying to be funny.

DR. IAN: People think you're funny because you're smart and your timing is great. Losing weight won't affect your delivery in any way. Don't be afraid of weight-loss success because you've wrapped your identity around the weight. When people see the new you, they'll not only see a funny comedian but one who looks good also.

JL went on to reach his goal and even exceed it. Not only did his audiences still find him funny, but his national visibility increased tremendously, and fans across the country flooded his box with congratulatory e-mails. More than a year later he had kept every pound off. Every time I see him on television I think about our conversation and how just a minor mental adjustment changed his life forever.

Take pride in your weight loss and enjoy the rewards that it brings. Your physique might change and your wardrobe will change, but your core values will still stay the same. Don't run away from success. Learn to embrace it.

VISUALIZE THE THIN YOU

I first heard of the concept of visualization when chatting with a sports psychologist who was sitting next to me in the green room at NBC. I was interested in his take on what separated the great players from the good ones. He talked about his personal experiences working with thousands of athletes who wanted to be not just good at what they did but to master the game. Then he talked about some of the greatest names in golf—players such as Jack Nicklaus and Sam Snead—whose ability to focus on the course had won them more championships than anyone in the history of the game.

This is how Jack Nicklaus described, in his book *Golf My Way*, his positive thinking and visualization before swinging the club:

> I never hit a shot, not even in practice, without having a very sharp, in-focus picture of it in my head. It's like a color movie. First I see the ball where I want it to finish, nice and white and sitting up high on bright green grass. Then the scene quickly changes and I see the ball going there: its path, trajectory and shape, even its behavior on landing. Then there is a sort of fade out and the next scene shows me making the kind of swing that will turn the previous images into reality.

The legendary golfer Sam Snead would often talk about how he painted a picture in the sky of the shot he planned to hit. Even golf phenom Tiger Woods has openly discussed how integral mental toughness and focus have been in his staggering success: "Mental toughness, I think you could put it into words," he said. "It's stuff like you never give up. You never give in to anything. You never accept anything but the best from yourself. You can always push to get better."

Visualization is commonly used in sports. It's the art of creating a mental model or image of an event or situation before it actually happens. It's not just seeing the image but actually *feeling* the experience that makes a difference. Experts in the field of visualization believe that there is an actual physiological response within the body when someone correctly visualizes. Thoughts and images can establish neurological patterns, and these patterns can cause muscular reactions that lead to the desired response. According to Performance Media, a company that specializes in visualization exercises:

> Vivid and detailed visualization can create a powerful effect on the body. Vividness and precision in visualizations create a physical sensation in the body. This kinesthetic or "feeling" component of the visualization is of vital importance. Feeling and sensing the experience as it is being pictured signify that the muscles and nervous system are strongly imprinted by the visualization.

I believe that visualization can be equally effective outside of the sports realm. People trying to lose weight can benefit greatly by making this a daily part of their regimen. Seeing and feeling yourself already achieving your goal can make your brain believe that actually attaining that goal is possible.

No single visualization technique is far superior to all others. You should choose one you're comfortable with and that proves to be effective for you. I have taken bits and pieces from various strategies and melded them together in a technique that I like to call "vivid animation."

I think of visualization as creating a colorful movie. The key, however, is to see the movie not through someone else's eyes but your own. Visualization should always be a first-person experience and not a third-person experience. Once you close your eyes, the darkness should immediately fill up with colorful images. Make your short movie as vivid as possible. You want all your senses to be involved. If you're standing near the ocean, smell the damp salt. If you're standing near a road, hear the car tires rolling over the pavement. If you're standing in your bathing suit on a hot day, feel the sun bead sweat on your skin. Whatever the scene you're part of, make sure you observe and feel all of it.

Let's say you want to lose 20 pounds. Try to see and *feel* yourself 20 pounds lighter. Imagine standing in a dressing room surrounded by new clothes you want to try on after losing weight. See the drab color of the walls in contrast to the bright colors of the clothes hanging on the hooks. Hear the chattering of the customers in the department store as well as the opening and closing of doors of the other dressing rooms. Smell the newness of the clothes and the age of the carpet. Take your clothes off and see the physical changes in your body. Your stomach doesn't bulge as it used to, and your legs actually have definition along the muscle planes. The back of your arms don't jiggle but instead are more firm.

You pick up a pair of jeans—two sizes smaller than what you've been wearing the last four months. You move the hangtags so that they're not in the way, and you lift your first leg into the jeans, then the second leg. You slowly pull them up your legs, and they feel more snug as they run over your thighs and settle around your waist. This is a nice feeling—snug but not too tight, formfitting but not transparent. Face the mirror and admire your physique and how great those jeans look and feel on your new body.

This is just one scenario, but there are thousands you can create to visualize your weight-loss success. Seeing and feeling a thinner you can actually create neurological patterns that spur muscle responses that lead to behaviors that bring about weight loss. Some people may want to visualize what they look like in a bathing suit, while others may choose to visualize a thirty-minute exercise session and the gratifying exhaustion they'll feel after completing their workout. You don't always have to visualize the same scenario; switch them depending on what you want to focus your mind on at the present time.

To perform your visualization I recommend finding a quiet area where you won't be interrupted or easily distracted. Spend 15 to 20 minutes every day visualizing some part of your journey. That should be enough to sharpen your mental focus and develop those neurological patterns that will eventually lead you to success. Occasionally, you might visualize the journey all the way to the end, but more frequently focus on smaller parts of the journey.

Work Box

LIST FOUR WAYS YOU WILL ACKNOWLEDGE YOUR WEIGHT LOSS DURING THE
COURSE OF THE JOURNEY:

1. _____

2. _____

3. _____

4. _____

LIST FIVE GOALS OR EVENTS THAT YOU WANT TO HAPPEN:

1. _____

2. _____

3. _____

4. _____

5. _____

VISUALIZATION OF YOUR GOALS—AT LEAST 15 TO 20 MINUTES EVERY DAY.

LIST THREE BIG-PERSON THINGS YOU DO THAT YOU CAN CHANGE:

1. _____

2. _____

3. _____

Visualization will not make what you want automatically happen. Tiger Woods still needs to practice for hours hitting golf balls and honing his skills on the course. You will still have to put the work in—choosing and eating the right foods, exercising with the necessary intensity for the right amount of time—to ultimately achieve your goals. But visualization can help you achieve those goals faster.

BONUS

S.M.A.R.T.E.R. EXERCISE

One of the biggest mistakes dieters make is refusing to exercise. Regardless of what food plan you're following, regular exercise should be part of your regimen. Let me explain why. Physical activity is an accelerant to weight loss. An accelerant is something that increases the speed of a process. Think about it in terms of a fire. You can start a fire by simply taking a match, striking it, and then setting the flame to an object. The fire will burn, but depending on the object and how large it is, it may take some time for the entire object to be burned. But if you throw an accelerant into the mix—such as kerosene, turpentine, or paint thinner—the fire will produce more heat, consume more quickly, burn at a higher temperature, and increase the spread of a fire. Exercise assists weight loss because it increases the speed and intensity at which calories are burned.

Studies overwhelmingly show that those who add regular exercise to calorie reduction not only lose more weight but keep the weight off the longest. Weight-loss professionals spend a great deal of time convincing skeptics that exercise is critical for optimal weight loss, but the health benefits are much broader than that. Exercise

- prevents or manages high blood pressure.
- lowers bad cholesterol (LDL) levels in your blood.
- increases the good cholesterol (HDL) levels in your blood.
- improves your mood and reduces feelings of depression and anxiety.
- improves your sex life.
- improves your sleep; you'll fall asleep faster and deepen your sleep.
- strengthens your heart and lungs.
- prevents chronic diseases such as type 2 diabetes, osteoporosis, and some types of cancer.
- adds years to your life.

Many people who don't regularly exercise don't know where to start. There are so many different forms and techniques of exercise that they get confused and do nothing. For weight loss, the two smartest types of exercise are cardiovascular activities and resistance training. Cardiovascular activities primarily benefit weight loss by increasing the number of calories that are burned. See the chart on the facing page. Your body needs energy to complete an exercise, whether it's riding a bike, walking on a treadmill, or swimming. The body gets this energy from three major sources: the food that you have recently eaten; glycogen (the stored form of glucose), which is found primarily in your muscles and liver; and fat. Remember, one of the major purposes of fat, beyond providing a layer of insulation for the body, is as a great source of energy. When your body needs energy—and moderate to intense cardiovascular exercise can create this need—it breaks down fat to release the stored energy.

Remember, if you're someone who has not been physically active recently, or you suffer from a medical problem, make sure you start off slowly and build gradually. Too many people jump right in and go full throttle and hurt themselves, because they tried to do too much too fast. It's good to push yourself when it comes to improving your exercise endurance, but pushing must be done thoughtfully and not to the extent that you put yourself at risk for injury.

"Resistance training" is the name of the category of exercises that work to increase muscle strength and endurance by doing repetitive exercises with weights, weight machines, or resistance bands. A common example is lifting dumbbells. It's a widespread misperception that resistance training is only for athletes, men, and those bodybuilder types who want to increase their muscularity dramatically. The truth, however, is that all of us can stand to benefit from resistance training, especially when trying to lose weight. Many women tell me they are nervous about resistance training because they don't want to be muscle-bound and appear masculine. This is something 99 percent of women will never have to worry about. It's not easy to develop the muscular physique of these body builders and competitive fitness contestants. They train rigorously for years and subject themselves to grueling workouts, long lifting sessions, and calorie-rich diets designed to build muscle, not lose weight. The resistance training you'll be doing will make your muscles come to life and give them tone, but it will not get you anywhere close to the bulging physiques of the zealous weight lifter.

ACTIVITY/CALORIES BURNED

ACTIVITY (ONE-HOUR DURATION)	WEIGHT OF PERSON AND CALORIES BURNED		
	160 pounds	200 pounds	240 pounds
Aerobics, high impact	511	637	763
Aerobics, low impact	365	455	545
Aerobics, water	292	364	436
Backpacking	511	637	763
Basketball game	584	728	872
Bicycling, < 10 mph, leisure	292	364	436
Bowling	219	273	327
Canoeing	256	319	382
Dancing, ballroom	219	273	327
Football, touch, flag, general	584	728	872
Golfing, carrying own clubs	329	410	491
Hiking	438	546	654
Ice skating	511	637	763
Jogging, 5 mph	584	728	872
Racquetball, casual, general	511	637	763
Rollerblading	913	1,138	1,363
Rope jumping	730	910	1,090
Rowing, stationary	511	637	763
Running, 8 mph	986	1,229	1,472
Skiing, cross-country	511	637	763
Skiing, downhill	365	455	545
Skiing, water	438	546	654
Softball or baseball	365	455	545
Stair treadmill	657	819	981
Swimming, laps	511	637	763
Tae kwon do	730	910	1,090
Tai chi	292	364	436
Tennis, singles	584	728	872
Volleyball	292	364	436
Walking, 2 mph	183	228	273
Walking, 3.5 mph	277	346	414

Source: Ainsworth, B.E.; Haskell, W.L.; Whitt, M.C.; Irwin, M.L.; Swartz, A.M.; Strath, S.J.; O'Brien, W.L.; Bassett, D.R. Jr.; Schmitz, K.H.; Emplaincourt, P.O.; Jacobs, D.R. Jr.; Leon, A.S.; Compendium of Physical Activities: An Update of Activity Codes and MET Intensities. *Medicine and Science in Sports and Exercise* 2000 Sep; 32(9 Suppl): S498–504.

You should consider resistance training for reasons beyond weight loss. The benefits are broad:

- Improves strength and balance
- Improves protection against physical injury
- Helps prevent/manage cardiovascular disease such as heart attacks, stroke, artery disease, and heart failure
- Improves diabetes management
- Assists cancer patients undergoing chemotherapy
- Prevents osteoporosis (bone thinning)
- Improves functioning and mobility in arthritis sufferers
- Improves lung function and rehabilitation for those suffering chronic conditions

Many people wonder why I recommend resistance training given that muscle weighs more than fat per unit volume. Their reasoning goes something like this: "If I'm burning away the fat and losing weight, won't adding muscle only put that weight back on?" To a minor degree new muscle will put some of that weight back on, but it is considered "good weight." One reason added muscle is good weight is that lean muscle mass actively helps burn calories overall even when you're not exercising.

Lean muscles are important for weight loss because they help boost your metabolism—the body's calorie-burning furnace. Muscles are high maintenance, and this is a good thing. They require a constant flow of energy and nutrition to keep them active and happy. This means that all those extra calories that might otherwise be sitting around waiting to be converted to fat are more likely to be burned by your muscles. The more lean muscle you develop, the more energy your muscles require, the more calories your furnace burns, and the greater your chance of losing weight.

A program that burns calories not only through cardiovascular exercise but also through resistance training and muscle development is optimal for weight loss. The program you decide to follow should take your personal preferences and capabilities into consideration. However, here is a recommended activity schedule you might want to consult as you begin a S.M.A.R.T.E.R. exercise program.

DAY 1	
35 minutes of cardio	15 minutes on treadmill*
	20 minutes on stationary bike
DAY 2	
30 minutes of cardio	15 minutes of power walking
15 minutes of resistance exercises	5 minutes of jumping rope
	10 minutes of walking stairs
	Resistance: leg presses, leg curls, hamstring curls
DAY 3	
Rest day	Rest
DAY 4	
35 minutes of cardio	20 minutes of rollerblading
	15 minutes of fast walking or jogging
DAY 5	
30 minutes of cardio	20 minutes on treadmill
20 minutes of resistance exercise	10 minutes on elliptical machine
	Resistance: chest presses, triceps extensions
DAY 6	
Rest day	Rest
DAY 7 (BONUS DAY)	
35 minutes of cardio or resistance	Since this is bonus day, choose your favorite exercises, whether cardio or resistance.

Note: You should strive for a moderate to intense level of effort while exercising. The times in this chart are just suggestions, and if you are capable and want to do more, by all means do so. If you are a beginner, then cut all times in half, and every two weeks try to add 2 minutes to your workout. If you have never been taught the proper safety techniques for exercising, seek professional supervision and instruction until you are proficient enough to exercise independently.

CHAPTER 6

Every Bite Counts

RELATIONSHIPS MATTER

What is your relationship to food? Do you eat because you're depressed and need comfort? When you're stressed, do you reach for that big bag of potato chips? Are you a social eater, someone who attends lots of functions that are centered around eating? Maybe you're like many I've counseled who have said that they are lonely and food is always a reliable friend.

Figuring out *your* relationship to food is critical for successful weight loss. So many of us eat and don't really understand why we're eating. We're not hungry, but we can't stop ourselves. We consume and aren't even aware of what we're consuming. It's called "mindless eating"—eating simply because the food is there. Eating is something to do, so we just reach into that bowl of trail mix and shovel handful after handful into our mouths as we watch TV or read the newspaper. It's almost as if the body has developed an eating reflex that is triggered not by hunger but by the availability of food.

Think about when you eat and why you eat. Do you follow a regular meal/snack schedule? Think about your hunger level when you eat. Are there times throughout the day that you're eating a snack or meal, and you're really not hungry? But it's lunch time or you're around others who are eating, so you join in. Identifying your eating triggers will give you a clearer picture of when you're eating out of necessity versus eating out of convenience.

FOOD IS FUEL

How you view food and its effects can go a long way in helping you improve your relationship and take better control of your eating. Our bodies are like cars with V-12 engines. We have the potential to run very hard and for long distances, but our performance is predicated on many variables. One of the most important variables is the type of gas that we put in our engines. Most manufacturers of luxury cars will explain that your vehicle will run best when consistently fed a diet of the highest octane gas. There are all types of reasons why they're right: Our luxury vehicles ride better and the engines last longer if we follow the manufacturer's suggestion to use premium unleaded gas.

The same is true of our bodies. Each of our organ systems—cardiovascular, respiratory, neurological, etc.—are like parts in our body's engine. They operate best and allow our entire body to function at its peak when fed the best fuel. Food is necessary fuel, and the higher its octane level, the harder and longer our bodies can run.

Often when I give a talk about obesity or nutrition, I ask the room, "How many of you indulge, at least every once in a while, in unhealthy foods that are high in calories and saturated fats and low in nutritional value—foods such as potato chips and pastries?" Hands are raised by almost everyone in the room, some more slowly than others, but all are raised when I subtly remind them of the need for honesty. Then I'll ask a follow-up question: "How many of you have ever put lemonade or water or dish detergent in your gas tank because you're low on money and gas prices are too high?" I typically get two responses: people looking at me as if I'd just landed from another planet or laughter at the absurdity of the idea. After the commotion has settled, I say, "So what you've just told me is that all of you are willing to put unhealthy fuel into your body but are not willing to put unhealthy fuel into your car even in desperate times. The well-being of your car outranks the well-being of your precious bodies." Invariably, a collective sigh of understanding sweeps across the room.

When you think of food as fuel that powers your body, you automatically want the best fuel possible. Vegetables, fruits, lean meats, and fish are the high-octane foods our bodies need for peak performance. These foods are low in calories and high in nutritional value, full of important nutrients, cancer fighters, protein, and fiber. Regardless of one's dieting philosophy, it is difficult to deny the overwhelming health benefits of these food categories. It will serve you well to make sure these foods dominate your consumption chart, unlike the foods we tend to eat for sheer pleasure or for convenience—something to quickly satisfy our hunger. See the chart on the next page.

Create your own consumption chart. Analyze everything you eat on a typical day. Don't immediately change the way you've been eating the last year just to make the chart look good. In order for this to work, you have to be honest and report your typical eating behavior. Once you've carved up your own chart and recorded the relative percentages of foods and beverages you eat, work on making sure the shaded part—the dominant part—is much bigger than the rest of the chart. This will mean that you're putting your focus on high-octane foods that will not only help you lose weight faster but provide you with better health protection and energy.

"EAT LIKE A KING FOR BREAKFAST, A PRINCE FOR LUNCH, AND A PAUPER FOR DINNER"

It's not just what you're eating but when you're eating that counts. Some people aren't necessarily eating the wrong things, but they're eating the wrong quantities of food at the wrong times. Continuing the car analogy, the one major difference between our body and our car is what happens to unused fuel. When you fill up your car's gas tank, the car is ready to travel at a moment's notice. If you park your car in the garage and don't use it for some time, the fuel will stay in the tank, ready to be put to use the minute you jump in the car and start the engine again. That is not the case with fuel—food—we put in our body's tank. If you load up your body with food and then don't move, the fuel stays there, but it doesn't stay accessible the way gas in a tank does. Instead, our bodies convert it and store it as fat, making fat our largest source of stored fuel. When you place physical demands on your body, the fuel comes from anything you might have recently eaten or from stores of energy in your muscles, but the biggest fuel source—and the most beneficial source for weight loss—is fat storage. Your body will take the fat and via several complicated processes break it down into energy that your body can instantly use.

This is why the timing of your food consumption is just as critical as what you eat. Eating a heavier meal in the morning means that you have the rest of

CONSUMPTION CHART

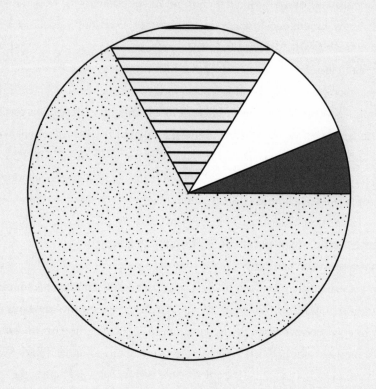

▦ Fruits, vegetables, lean meats, fish

⊟ Dairy

☐ Cakes, cookies, pastries,
candy, sweet beverages

■ Fatty meats, breads, grains

the day to burn off those calories. That's why pioneering nutritionist Adele Davis said you should eat like a king for breakfast and load up on the best fuel for both physical and mental power.

Eating like a prince for lunch is critical for several reasons. Depending on when you eat lunch, you are halfway or more through your workday. It's still important to have the proper fuel to get through the rest of the day productively. But it also means that you're getting closer to the evening when your activities typically wind down and you'll be going to sleep. This means you'll have less of an opportunity to burn fuel. Remember, any unused fuel will get converted to fat, so it's smart to eat a satisfying lunch but it's also important not to overdo it.

Dinner is the last meal of the day, which means your car is in the driveway and almost in the garage. While American eating habits mean that dinner is often the heaviest of our meals—the whole "steak and potatoes" routine—new medical research has taught us how harmful that way of thinking really is. Eating your heaviest meal closest to the time you go to sleep is a perfect recipe for weight gain. When you go to sleep, your metabolism—the body's internal calorie-burning furnace—slows down to almost nothing because the body is at rest. Once your metabolism slows down, all the fuel that hasn't been burned yet—dinner and even a late lunch—gets converted and stored as fat.

YOUR PERSONAL FOOD ANALYZER

Have you ever thought about why you eat certain foods? The no-brainer answers are: "Because I like them" and "They taste great." But there are other reasons, too. If you take a few minutes to think about them, you might be surprised. If you can figure out why you're eating certain foods, then you can figure out how to change your eating habits.

To create your personal food analyzer, take a blank sheet of paper. In the middle of the page, list the foods and beverages you consume most frequently— both healthy and unhealthy. Then on the left side of the page list the health benefits you might derive from eating nutritious food. On the right side of the page, list the emotional benefits you might derive from eating certain foods. Once you've formed your lists, it's time to make the connections. Draw lines from all the listed foods to the health benefits in the left column. Then, draw lines from

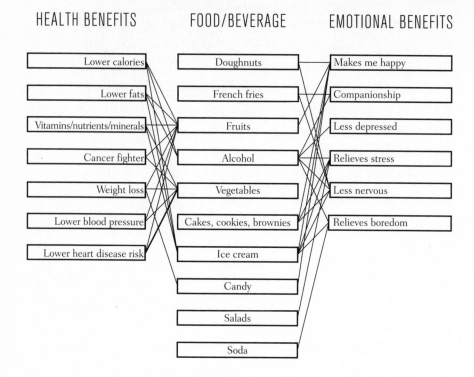

HEALTH BENEFITS	FOOD/BEVERAGE	EMOTIONAL BENEFITS
Lower calories	Doughnuts	Makes me happy
Lower fats	French fries	Companionship
Vitamins/nutrients/minerals	Fruits	Less depressed
Cancer fighter	Alcohol	Relieves stress
Weight loss	Vegetables	Less nervous
Lower blood pressure	Cakes, cookies, brownies	Relieves boredom
Lower heart disease risk	Ice cream	
	Candy	
	Salads	
	Soda	

the various food/beverage items to the emotional benefits in the right column. Look at the sample above to get a better idea of how to make a food analyzer. You'll probably add more foods or take some away when creating your analyzer. You can increase or decrease the list of emotions. What matters is that you take the time to think about your answers and report them honestly. Not being truthful won't hurt anyone but you.

Once your chart is complete, find the food/beverages that have the largest number of connections to the left-hand side of the chart. Those are the items you should be consuming in abundance. Now look at the right-hand side of the chart. Those items that have the most connections on this side of the chart represent emotional eating, foods that can be comforting and temporarily change your mood, but, as you can see, do not provide much in the way of health benefits.

EMOTIONAL EATING

How do you know if you're an emotional eater? It's not terribly difficult to figure out. If you eat in response to your feelings rather than to hunger, you are probably an emotional eater. Here's another way to figure it out. Answer yes to any of the questions below, and you are doing some emotional eating.

Do you eat because you're bored?

Do you find comfort in food?

When you're upset, sad, nervous, or lonely do you have specific food cravings?

Do you ever eat without even realizing you're doing it (mindless eating)?

Do you ever eat when you're not hungry but in response to your feelings?

Do you ever feel guilty after eating?

Why does emotional eating matter when you're trying to lose weight and take control of your eating? Emotional eating often leads to overeating. In fact, many studies suggest that as much as 75 percent of overeating is due to emotional eating. Food is like a drug for emotional eaters. It's a convenient way to medicate feelings of sadness, depression, loneliness, anxiety, guilt, and many others. If the overeating involved foods such as fruits and vegetables and other low-calorie fare, then there wouldn't be a negative impact on your weight loss. Unfortunately, the foods we reach for to feel better tend to be more fattening, sweeter, or saltier.

The good news is that there are ways to change your eating patterns.

BECOME A MINDFUL EATER

Too many of us don't pay attention to what we're eating or how we're eating—we're eating mindlessly. We are too distracted doing other things, whether it's watching television, working on our computer, or driving the car. Our attention is focused on everything else other than the food we're eating. It's this lack of focus that leads to poor eating habits. The optimal condition for eating meals is a quiet place away from any distractions where we can sit down and truly enjoy the taste of the food as well as the company of those eating with us. Give yourself enough time to eat, and stop trying to squeeze it in between appointments. Allowing yourself to focus on your food means a better appreciation for what and how much you're putting inside your body.

FIND OTHER WAYS TO COPE WITH YOUR EMOTIONS

Emotions, even negative ones, are not always a bad thing. There are circumstances that make us sad, and there are times we feel alone. It's okay sometimes to be disappointed in ourselves and others, and there are times when our stress level rises in response to certain situations. It's not the emotion itself that causes harm but our reaction to that emotion and how we deal with it that really matters. Coping with our emotions through food is unhealthy. Instead of reaching for that bag of potato chips when you're disappointed, try calling a friend and talking about what's bothering you. There are many simple coping strategies you can try that have nothing to do with food. Taking a peaceful walk, listening to music, reading an engaging book, or writing in your journal are all effective ways to ease stress or take the edge off disappointment without resorting to overeating. Find a strategy that works for you and go for it.

EXERCISE

The benefits of exercise are endless. You know that exercise burns calories, improves heart and lung function, and prevents obesity. But exercise can also be instrumental when trying to avoid emotional eating. It can relieve stress and anxiety as well as increase your energy level. Exercise also does something special by prompting the body to release endorphins into your bloodstream. Endorphins are chemicals that block pain signals from reaching your brain. These chemicals provide a "natural high," helping to alleviate anxiety and depression.

DON'T EXPECT PERFECTION

Striving for perfection can be a double-edged sword. We want to do our best and succeed, but when we don't hit the mark, we can become disappointed and in some cases depressed. This leads to poor responses such as trying to eat ourselves back to a positive mind-set. Accept that perfection is often elusive and, if not reached, does not signal failure. Lofty goals are admirable but must be accompanied by a healthy dose of reality. Expecting perfection can be a setup for failure and all the poor behavioral responses that come with it.

EAT THE RIGHT FOODS

If you simply must indulge in foods during times of emotional crisis, then at the very least reach for the foods that come with health benefits. The comfort foods we typically reach for—high in calories and sugar—cause blood sugar spikes and lows. This is exactly what you want to avoid when trying to lose weight or prevent weight gain. There are foods, however, that don't cause these spikes and lows: raw vegetables, whole fruits, whole-grain breads and cereals, popcorn without butter. The wrong foods at the wrong time might seem effective for a quick fix, but they will only create long-term problems that you will be forced to address in the future.

CONTROL YOUR ENVIRONMENT

If the unhealthy food isn't there, you can't eat it. Why tempt yourself unnecessarily? Clean out your cabinets and refrigerator and toss the chocolates, chips, sodas, and ice cream, so that even though you may want to turn to these foods for comfort when you are facing an emotional crisis, they won't be available. Too many people say that they are strong enough to resist the urge, yet they often hold off as long as they can and then eventually give in, knowing the only thing that separates them from resolving their emotional conflict is a walk to the kitchen. Remove the temptation, and you'll remove the possibility of doing what you're not supposed to do.

SMALL SUBSTITUTIONS CAN MAKE A BIG DIFFERENCE

In your effort to eat smarter and not waste calories, it's important to understand that just by making simple substitutions you can save calories and not give up taste. The idea that "every bite counts" doesn't just apply to bigger items such as meats and sweets but also to smaller ones that can have a real impact on your overall plan. While successful dieting is definitely more than just counting calories, saving them wherever you can gives you an advantage. What you slather on your sandwich or drizzle over your salad can make the difference—a couple of hundred calories' worth. To help you save precious calories, study the chart on the next page. It lists simple substitutions you might make and the amount of calories you'll save by doing so.

Smart Substitutions Chart

INSTEAD OF	TRY	CALORIES SAVED (1 SERVING)
Guacamole	Salsa	46
Carrot cake (3 oz)	Gingerbread	51
Mayonnaise (1 tsp)	Mustard	54
New England clam chowder	Manhattan clam chowder	60
Potato chips (1 oz)	Unbuttered popcorn	60
Whole milk (1 cup)	Skim milk	60
Ranch salad dressing (2 tbsp)	Raspberry vinaigrette	68
Tartar sauce (1 tbsp)	Lemon juice	70
Regular potato chips (1 oz)	Baked potato chips	90
Peking/hoisin sauce (3 oz)	Oyster sauce	99
Soft drink (1 can)	Water	100
Hershey chocolate bar	Nestlé rich chocolate hot cocoa	105
Cinnamon raisin bagel	Cinnamon raisin English muffin	106
Buttered popcorn (1 cup)	Air-popped popcorn	108
Pudding (1 cup)	Sugar-free applesauce	108
5th Avenue candy bar	Fig bars (3)	115
Bagel with cream cheese (1 tbsp)	Apple slices with peanut butter	119
Café latte	Hot tea	122
Ground beef (4 oz)	Ground turkey	132
Cream of chicken soup	Chicken noodle soup	140
Cinnamon Pop-Tart (2)	Large graham crackers (4)	140
Cheddar cheese (1 cup)	Mozzarella cheese	141

INSTEAD OF	TRY	CALORIES SAVED (1 SERVING)
Ice cream (½ cup)	Nonfat frozen yogurt	153
Hollandaise sauce (1 cup)	White wine sauce	160
Ricotta cheese (1 cup)	Low-fat cottage cheese	172
Chocolate chip cookies (5)	Vanilla wafers	200
Flaked coconut (1 cup)	Diced pineapple	265
Cream (1 cup)	Evaporated milk	300
Veggie pizza (2 slices)	No-cheese veggie pizza	314
Sour cream (1 cup)	Plain yogurt	343
Nachos with the works	Tortilla chips and salsa	414
Fettuccine Alfredo (16 oz)	Spaghetti with tomato sauce	426
Chocolate (1 cup)	Cocoa	492

Work Box

1. Identify your eating triggers.

2. Create your consumption chart.

3. Create your personal food analyzer.

CHAPTER 7

Reward Yourself

One of the critical components of setting goals and working hard to attain them is what awaits you on the other side of success. This is the fun chapter—figuring out how to reward yourself for all your dedication and hard work. Thinking about your rewards is not as simple as you might think. It's not just saying, "If I lose 40 pounds I'm going to buy myself a new TV." No, setting your reward structure is just as critical as setting your goals; so take the time to be reasonable and S.M.A.R.T.E.R about your choices.

One of the important features of the reward system is that *you* make the choices. It's important that the rewards are something you have chosen because you truly want them and that they inspire you to complete your task. Some people reward themselves with new clothes, others jewelry, and some with relaxing vacations. There is no such thing as a preset list of the right and wrong rewards. What makes the reward right is that you have chosen it, you can afford it, and it's of enough sentimental or material value that you will stay inspired and work hard to reach your goal.

Remember when you set your weight-loss goals? We talked about setting the ultimate goal—the number you wanted to reach at the end of the weight-loss portion of your journey. But we also talked about setting smaller goals that will add up to the big goal. The same is true for setting your rewards. You can have a big reward such as a weeklong trip to Paris. But along the way you will be reaching smaller milestones, maybe losing 3 or 5 pounds every few weeks, so they, too, should be rewarded in some way.

While the type of rewards is ultimately your choice, they should have certain characteristics.

Attainable. Don't set rewards that are dreams and you have no realistic chance of acquiring them. Reality in your reward setting is just as critical as it was in your goal setting. Making unrealistic reward plans is one of the biggest mistakes that people commit. For example, promising yourself that you'll purchase a Mercedes when you reach your ultimate goal when you know very well that your income and budget won't financially allow you to purchase such an expensive car is irresponsible and potentially counterproductive. If you know that you really can't attain your reward, then you are much less likely to work to reach your goal. In the back of your mind you know that there's no *real* reward waiting to meet the results of your hard work.

Graduated. Your rewards should grow in importance to match the growth of your goals. If your first milestone is 3 pounds of a 30-pound ultimate goal, don't make the reward for that first 3-pound milestone a new computer then make the reward for the 15-pound milestone a new pair of jeans. This is upside down and won't provide the encouragement to keep going to the next level. Your drive to reach the next milestone should increase along with your weight loss, thus allowing the reward system to truly be part of your inspiration for success. Set your rewards on a sliding scale.

Motivational. What good is a reward if it doesn't motivate? The reward, whether at the beginning of the journey or at the end, must goad you into action. You must want this reward enough that it keeps you committed to your plan even through rough spots and challenges. If you find yourself asking whether toughing it out during the journey is worth it, then you might not have the appropriate rewards in place. Carefully select those rewards that you want badly enough to keep you working hard toward your goals.

Unique. Making your reward something that is as mundane as a T-shirt will do little in the way of encouraging you to work hard for that next goal. The reward should be unique enough that it holds a special meaning and is not something you would simply acquire anytime you had the slightest inkling. Rewards, whether a visit to an art exhibit, dinner at your favorite restaurant, or a new electronic gadget, are most helpful when they are extraordinary.

It is important to remember the true purpose of the reward and to make sure the reward does not overshadow the bigger goal of losing weight and becoming healthier. No reward, regardless of how expensive or exciting, should eclipse the luster and importance of the primary mission of your journey. This is one of the dangers that can emerge with a reward system, but it is completely avoidable if you take this into account when setting up your reward structure.

Below is an example of how one might set up a goal and companion reward structure:

GOAL	REWARD
3 pounds	A shirt you've been dying to buy
8 pounds	A long afternoon at your favorite museum
10 pounds	Dinner at your favorite restaurant
14 pounds	A weekend of total relaxation
20 pounds	A day spa treatment
23 pounds	A new digital camera
27 pounds	A new handbag or briefcase
30 pounds	A really nice piece of jewelry

Rewarding weight-loss milestones makes sense, but there are other things you should reward along the journey. Celebrating your behavioral changes is equally important. The positive changes you make are critical in helping you reach your goals, and thus they should also be part of the reward system. Which behavioral changes you reward are based on your preferences, but some you might consider include sticking to your chosen plan for a certain period of time, not having thoughts of failure, keeping up your exercise schedule for two weeks, eating only a portion of a bag of chips and not the entire bag, resisting those fattening late-night desserts, and choosing water for your meal more often than you choose soda.

It is important to remember that beyond the numeric goal, the biggest achievement you can make along the journey is a pattern of positive behavioral changes that will last a lifetime. There should come a point when you are no longer following a diet but rather simply *living*, making dietary and physical activity choices that are smart, sustainable, and prevent weight gain and other unhealthy outcomes. Thoughts are really our guides as they serve as the engines for our actions. The more positive your thoughts, the more likely you are to be successful. The more you acknowledge and reward yourself for even the smallest of successes, the greater the likelihood that you will reach even greater successes. The numbers on the scale might excite you, but once you realize that you have gained better control of your life through making healthier choices, you will be inspired to continue in that positive direction and never to turn back.

CHAPTER 8

The Modular Eating Plan

Here it is! It's time to take all you've learned in previous chapters and put it to work. The modular eating plan will help you lose weight *and* become healthier. It's not just another quick-fix diet that makes unrealistic promises. It will teach you how to choose the highest octane fuel for your engine and reach peak performance. There is no such thing as "one plan fits all," so don't be afraid to make some substitutions or adjustments if you're allergic to certain foods or have a medical condition that prevents you from eating some of the foods on the plan. "I don't like certain foods" is not an excuse. Open your mind and palate to new foods and tastes. You might come to enjoy foods you had convinced yourself you didn't like.

The modular eating plan is broken up into smaller modules—four-day segments—that change the type and quantity of food you'll eat. I do this for several reasons. First, like our marathon runner in Chapter 2, it's to your advantage to focus on smaller segments of the race rather than the entire marathon. It's much easier to think about what you'll be eating (and not eating) over a four-day span rather than thinking about what you'll be eating (and not eating) for several weeks. Second, the modular eating plan allows you to work a variety of foods into your diet so that you don't get bored eating the same food.

Third, these modules will be effective in pushing your body to lose weight because the variety of the types and amount of food you consume along with your exercise will keep the body off-kilter. This experience of being off-kilter is important because it means your body never gets a chance to grow accustomed to the food or the exercise, thus the body is constantly surprised by what you eat and the physical activities you demand it accomplish. This is the optimal state for weight loss, especially as you aim to reach those smaller goals on the way to the ultimate goal. The more your body needs to adjust to its environment, the more energy it will expend, and the more calories it will need to burn to provide that energy. Burning more calories leads to weight loss. As these dieting modules force continual adjustments within your body, it will likely take you longer to reach a weight-loss plateau. And when you do hit one, you'll bust through it faster than if you stuck to the same eating/exercise regimen.

Another effective aspect of the program is its simplicity. Long, complicated eating plans tend to confuse and frustrate dieters who try to follow them. Don't overthink the plan. I have laid it out for you in modules that consist of simple food lists. Follow the modules, and you will master not only the plan but the lifestyle changes that will lead to a longer, slimmer, and healthier life.

Special Note: You are allowed two 8-ounce cups of coffee per day.

The INDUCTION Module

This is the first module that you will follow. Except for the TRANSITION module, which comes next, the rest of the modules do not have to be followed in order, but it's important to start with INDUCTION no matter how much you have to lose. The purpose of the INDUCTION module is to help remove some of the toxins that have accumulated in your body from not making the healthiest food decisions. It will clear your body and mind for the changes that come next. INDUCTION is written as a four-day plan, but you can make it longer if you like by simply repeating some of the days. However, to do IN-DUCTION right, you *must* complete four days. The INDUCTION module gives you invigorating, extremely healthy foods that not only mop up the toxins floating around in your body but naturally increase your energy. The quantities listed are the maximum amounts that can be consumed for that day. It doesn't mean, however, that you have to eat all the food listed; you can eat less if you desire. Remember, eat enough to satisfy your hunger, but don't eat until you're stuffed. Distribute the food throughout the day, but make sure you front load your meals by eating most of the food during the earlier part of the day.

You might need to make some substitutions because you're allergic to certain foods or you can't obtain the foods easily. (This shouldn't happen often because the foods are simple, inexpensive, and can be found in most restaurants and local grocery stores.) If you substitute, make S.M.A.R.T. substitutions and don't substitute a 12-ounce steak for a 4-ounce serving of fish. A major part of what you're trying to accomplish during INDUCTION is learning how to make S.M.A.R.T.E.R. choices naturally, without having someone tell you what works and what doesn't.

Day 1

2 cups of coffee (8 oz per cup). Limit sugar to 1 packet and cream or milk to 1 tsp per cup.

2 cups of raw or cooked green leafy vegetables (such as spinach, collard greens, kale, Swiss chard, arugula, lettuce, celery)

1 cup of freshly squeezed lemonade with no more than 1 tbsp of sugar

10 grams of psyllium husk (1 tbsp of psyllium husk powder added to water or lemonade; or try a bowl of psyllium-enriched cereal with no more than ½ cup of low-fat, reduced-fat, fat-free, skim, or soy milk)

4 servings of fruit: 1 medium apple, 1 medium banana, 1 medium pear, ⅔ cup of blueberries, ½ cup of raspberries, ½ cup of strawberries, etc.

One 6-oz low-fat or fat-free yogurt *without* "fruit on the bottom." Add your own fresh fruit if you like.

1 medium-size (2 cups) green garden salad, vegetables only—no bacon bits, croutons, eggs, etc.—plus 3 tbsp of fat-free or low-fat dressing

1 cup of cooked beans, chickpeas, lentils, or other legumes (but no baked beans)

1½ cups of cooked brown rice (measured after cooking)

Unlimited plain water (seltzer water is an option). Be sure to drink 1 cup of water before each meal.

EXERCISE

40 minutes of cardio

NOTE: Always try to drink 1 cup of water before eating each meal. Water is important not just for flushing out the kidneys and helping to eliminate toxins from your body, but it helps make you feel full on less food. Drinking water before eating helps take up some of the limited space in the stomach and causes expansion. When you eat solid food after drinking water, the stomach has less room to expand and sends a signal to the brain that you are full, cutting off your drive to eat more.

You might not be able to do 40 minutes of consecutive cardio exercise, and that's just fine. Go ahead and break it up into segments. You might do 20 minutes, take a rest, and then do the second 20 minutes. You can break it up and do it anytime throughout the day. Just make sure to get in a total of 40 minutes of cardio work. As you build your endurance, you'll be able to do more exercise continuously until you can do the entire 40-minute period at one time.

S.M.A.R.T.E.R. Choice Box

PSYLLIUM

Plantago psyllium is a plant native to West Pakistan and India. The stalks of the plant contain tiny seeds that are also called psyllium. These seeds are covered by husks, the part of the plant that is used in foods such as psyllium-fortified cereals. This husk is important because it is a source of water-soluble fiber, the kind of fiber that you also find in common grains such as oat and barley. Psyllium, however, is a more potent fiber source. The effect of soluble fiber in 1 tablespoon of psyllium is equal to 14 tablespoons of oat bran. Psyllium mops up various toxins and helps to clear them out.

Psyllium is also part of the "soluble fiber" food category that can help lower cholesterol, according to the American Heart Association. Most recommend a maximum daily dosage of 10 grams. Psyllium has long been used as a chief ingredient in "bulk laxatives." It can be purchased and used in powder form. There are some side effects, however, that you should be aware of when taking psyllium. They include but aren't limited to difficulty swallowing; frequent bowel movements; gas; skin irritation, rash, or itching; and intestinal blockage.

Never take psyllium dry but instead mix it with 6–8 ounces of liquid, preferably water.

Day 2

2 cups of coffee (8 oz per cup). Limit sugar to 1 packet and cream or milk
 to 1 tsp per cup.

2 scrambled eggs or egg whites (¼ cup of chopped vegetables optional)

1 cup of freshly squeezed juice

3 servings of fruit: 1 medium apple, 1 medium banana, 1 medium pear, ½
 cup of blueberries, ½ cup of raspberries, ½ cup of strawberries, etc.

1 large-size (3 cups) green garden salad with watercress; vegetables only—no
 bacon bits, croutons, eggs, etc.—plus 3 tbsp of fat-free or low-fat dressing

2 cups of green leafy vegetables (such as spinach, collard greens, kale,
 Swiss chard, arugula, lettuce, celery)

1 cup of vegetable juice from the cooked vegetables

1 cup of cooked brown rice (measured after cooking)

EXERCISE

40 minutes of cardio

NOTE: Use your servings of fruit strategically. Eat them to fill the "holes" between the meals—snacks. Also, try eating fruit with the skin. The skin makes
you chew longer, which means you'll eat it more slowly. The skin also contains lots of the nutrients such as fiber.

Day 3

2 cups of coffee (8 oz per cup). Limit sugar to 1 packet and cream or milk
   to 1 tsp per cup.

One 6-oz low-fat or fat-free yogurt *without* "fruit on the bottom." Add your
   own fresh fruit if you like.

3 servings of fruit: 1 medium apple, 1 medium banana, 1 medium pear, ½
   cup of blueberries, ½ cup of raspberries, ½ cup of strawberries, etc.

2 cups of green leafy vegetables (such as spinach, collard greens, kale,
   Swiss chard, arugula, lettuce, celery)

1 cup of freshly squeezed lemonade (with no more than 1 tbsp of sugar)

10 grams of psyllium husk (1 tbsp of psyllium husk powder added to water
   or lemonade; or try a bowl of psyllium-enriched cereal with no more
   than ½ cup of low-fat, reduced-fat, fat-free, skim, or soy milk)

1 medium-size (2 cups) green garden salad, vegetables only—no bacon
   bits, croutons, eggs, etc.—plus 3 tbsp of fat-free or low-fat dressing

1 cup of cooked beans, chickpeas, lentils, or other legumes (but no baked
   beans)

1 cup of cabbage soup (see recipe on page 184)

Unlimited plain water. Be sure to drink 1 cup of water before each meal.

EXERCISE

40 minutes of cardio

Day 4

FRUIT/VEGGIE DAY

Unlimited fruit of any kind (at least 3 servings)

1 cup of green tea or regular tea

1 large-size (3 cups) green garden salad; add garlic, and you can also add 3 oz of walnuts, Brazil nuts, cashew nuts, almonds, or sunflower seeds; no other toppings other than vegetables; 3 tbsp of fat-free or low-fat dressing

1 cup of freshly squeezed carrot juice (substitution allowed: freshly squeezed pear, apple, or orange juice)

10 grams of psyllium husk (1 tablespoon of psyllium husk powder added to water or lemonade; or try a bowl of psyllium-enriched cereal with no more than ½ cup of low-fat, reduced-fat, fat-free, skim, or soy milk)

2 cups of cooked brown rice (measured after cooking)

1 cup of cabbage soup (see recipe on page 184)

2 servings of cooked or raw vegetables

Unlimited plain water

EXERCISE

Rest day

Your body needs time to recover and strengthen. A rest day is designed to give you that time. If you still feel the need for a period of timed physical activity, however, try to do something such as playing tennis, walking around your neighborhood, playing basketball, or swimming. Try an activity that will give you the benefit of burning calories but is also fun and doesn't feel as if it's an "exercise chore."

NOTE: This day is meant to be a fruits and vegetables day only with the exception of 2 cups of cooked brown rice. You're also allowed to have 3 tbsp

(continued)

of low-fat or fat-free dressing per salad. This will be the last day of detox. Resist the urge to add other foods because it's important to keep this day as pure as possible. There will be plenty of opportunity in future modules for you to have many of the foods that weren't included in this module.

The TRANSITION Module

Congratulations on completing INDUCTION. Your body should feel cleansed and revitalized by the powerful foods you've eaten over the last four days. You now know that even if you're a meat eater, these four days have made you feel sharper, more energized, and slimmer. The purpose of the next module is to reintroduce foods into your meal plan, but not to go overboard. Part of the module system is teaching you how to make better food and beverage choices while at the same time you are learning to be comfortable with these choices and really enjoying them. No plan will work if it's not sustainable over the long term, and you consider it a chore to eat the foods because you don't like them. Or, worse, you feel you haven't eaten after a meal on the plan because you've been deprived of what you think a meal should look like. By going through modules, you are rewiring your body and brain as it relates to food. You must be patient and open to allow the process to take hold and change to occur. **THE 4 DAY DIET** really works, so let go of any lingering negativity or doubt.

The TRANSITION module is very simple. Study the food list. All four days are identical in terms of food intake and exercise. This is done on purpose. Try to avoid substitutions unless absolutely necessary. Once you have completed TRANSITION, you can use the other modules in your order of preference. And don't forget about exercise. Physical activity is critical, not just for your ability to lose the most weight possible, but for other health-boosting properties. The TRANSITION module is your bridge to the future. Think about this over the next four days as your mind and body prepare for the excitement—and hard work—that awaits.

Follow This TRANSITION Module for 4 Days

2 cups of coffee (8 oz per cup). Limit sugar to 1 packet and cream or milk to 1 tsp per cup.

1 cup of carrots, raw preferred but cooked is also fine

1 cup of sliced cucumbers with fat-free dressing (2 tbsp max)

1 cup of berries (any kind)

1 apple

1 pear

1 cup of cooked beans, chickpeas, lentils, or other legumes (but *no* baked beans)

One 4-oz serving of fish or chicken or turkey (no skin, no fried)

1 medium-size (2 cups) green garden salad, vegetables only—no bacon bits, croutons, eggs, etc.—plus 3 tbsp of fat-free or low-fat dressing

Unlimited plain water (at least 6 cups per day)

1 diet soda

2 snacks (see snacks list on page 139)

NOTE: These are the daily allowances. You can eat less, but not more. You *must* stick to the items on the menu. Eat only what you need. Try not to eat everything on the list. Keep a checklist of what you eat.

EXERCISE

Day 1: 40 minutes of cardio

Day 2: Two 30-minute cardio sessions—one in the a.m. and one in the p.m.

Day 3: Rest

Day 4: 40 minutes of cardio

Variety is important in all of the modules, so make sure you mix it up wherever you can. For example, try different berries each day. Also, instead of having four continuous days of fish or meat, try to alternate between fish and meat and the types that you eat.

Exercise is non-negotiable.

S.M.A.R.T.E.R. Choice Box

LEGUMES

Legumes are a class of vegetables that includes beans, peas, and lentils. These vegetables are extremely versatile in how they can be prepared and are some of the most nutritious foods you can include in your eating plan. They are typically low in fat, contain no cholesterol, and provide a high quantity of folate, potassium, iron, and magnesium. For those seeking more protein in their diet, legumes are a great source, and some might even consider them a healthier substitute for protein-rich red meat that contains a lot more fat and cholesterol.

Examples of legumes include but aren't limited to the following:

- Adzuki beans
- Anasazi beans
- Black beans
- Black-eyed peas
- Broad beans (fava beans)
- Butter beans
- Calico beans
- Cannellini beans
- Chickpeas (garbanzo beans)
- Edamame
- Fava beans
- Great Northern beans
- Italian beans
- Kidney beans
- Lentils
- Lima beans
- Mung beans
- Navy beans
- Pinto beans
- Soy beans, including black soy beans (also known as soy nuts)
- Split peas
- White beans

Make sure you avoid beans that are canned with sugar and/or lard.

The PROTEIN STRETCH Module

Before embarking on a run, trained athletes will engage in a regimen of stretching and other warm-up exercises. Preparation gets the muscles and other soft tissues loosened to prevent injury during the main event. Runners who might cramp in the middle of the race or complain of lower back and leg tightness will often blame a poor pre-run warm-up routine. The night before the big race, many marathoners "carb load"; in other words, they eat lots of pasta and other high-carb foods to store energy for the next day's run. The four-day PROTEIN STRETCH delivers the dieter's version of the same concept. But instead of carbs, we're going to load up on protein in this module.

The Institute of Medicine recommends that adults get a minimum of 0.8 gram of protein per day for every kilogram of body weight. That level of protein was selected to prevent the body from slowly breaking down its own tissues. For example, a 160-pound person (72.6 kg) should consume at least 58 grams of protein on a daily basis, which is the equivalent of eating two 4-ounce hamburger patties.

Our food environment is abundant in protein. There are readily available animal and vegetable sources. The best animal sources are fish and poultry. Other great sources include beans, nuts, and whole grains. The PROTEIN STRETCH module has been constructed so that you don't have to worry about performing any complex calculations. I have already done that for you. Just pay close attention to the food/drink list and the quantities that are listed. It is unwise not to eat enough protein, but it's also unwise to overconsume protein. Protein can be a key to weight loss if you consume it responsibly and choose the best sources of this powerful nutrient.

Follow This PROTEIN STRETCH Module for 4 Days

2 cups of coffee (8 oz per cup). Limit sugar to 1 packet and cream or milk to 1 tsp per cup.

2 scrambled eggs or egg whites (optional: add ¼ cup of chopped vegetables, tsp of oil for cooking)

1 strip of turkey bacon (substitution allowed: 1 small turkey sausage link)

1 small protein shake (200 calories or less)

2 servings of fruit (such as 1 medium apple and 1 medium banana)

1 cup of raw veggies (such as carrots, celery, red/yellow bell peppers, tomatoes)

1 sandwich (4 oz turkey, chicken, or lean sirloin; avoid white bread; 1 tbsp of low-fat mayo or mustard allowed)

1 cup of beans or other legumes

1 cup of brown rice (measured after cooking)

2 servings of cooked veggies

Unlimited plain water

EXERCISE

30 minutes of cardio

20 minutes of light weights such as 5–10-pound dumbbells (resistance training)

NOTE: You will be following this module for four days. As always, variety is a good way to keep yourself engaged and prevent boredom. Alternate items each day where possible. For example, the fruit, raw veggies, sandwich, beans/legumes, and cooked veggies can be different for each of the four days. If you want to eat the same thing all four days, you're certainly allowed to do that, but switch it up if you find yourself losing enthusiasm for the food.

The SMOOTH Module

Have you missed that burger or pasta or pizza or french fries? Well, you won't miss them much longer. The SMOOTH module is meant to give you some of your favorites without overindulging. If you balance your diet properly and eat bigger portions of the healthy foods, you can eat almost anything you want and enjoy the experience. Most people will be shocked that I'm giving you permission to eat things such as fries, burgers, and pizza, but I believe in being realistic. To think that someone is going to swear off these foods and never eat them again is ridiculous. I want you to get a taste of these foods but enjoy them in a moderate, reasonable way. There's almost no food in and of itself that is bad—it's only an excessive amount that is a problem.

The purpose of SMOOTH is to give you a taste of the old and a greater appreciation of the new. While I strongly recommend that you *reduce* fried foods, creamy sauces, and high-carb dishes such as white pasta to a minimum, it is okay for you to indulge periodically. I want you to really enjoy what you're eating and to realize that there is an infinite number of food combinations that are tasty and gratifying if you're willing to experiment. When nothing is off limits, you may find your choices become naturally wise ones.

Your body has made great strides throughout the last couple of modules. Don't give it all back by suddenly eating out of control. That's not what the SMOOTH module is all about. Enjoy what you eat but remember that every bite still counts.

Day 1

2 scrambled eggs or egg whites (optional: add ¼ cup of chopped vegetables; 1 tsp of oil for cooking)

1 piece of whole wheat or multigrain toast with butter

½ cup of blueberries

½ cup of strawberries

1 medium-size (2 cups) green garden salad, vegetables only—no bacon bits, croutons, eggs, etc.—plus 3 tbsp of fat-free or low-fat dressing

1 cup of cooked beans, chickpeas, lentils, or other legumes (but no baked beans)

2 medium slices of pizza (no bacon/sausage/pepperoni toppings; remember, you don't have to eat the full 2 slices, just eat until you aren't hungry). Substitutions allowed: 1 cup of pasta with tomato-based sauce—avoid cream sauce; 4-oz hamburger or veggie burger on a bun with a small order of french fries; 1 medium-size hot dog on a bun; 4 oz of fish; 4 oz of chicken (no skin, no fried).

One 100-calorie snack (see snacks list on page 139)

2 servings of cooked or raw veggies

1 cup of flavored water

Unlimited plain water

EXERCISE

1 hour total:

40 minutes of cardio

20 minutes of light weights (resistance training)

Day 2

2 cups of coffee (8 oz per cup). Limit sugar to 1 packet and cream or milk
    to 1 tsp per cup.

One 6-oz low-fat or fat-free yogurt *without* "fruit on the bottom." Add your
    own fresh fruit if you like.

1 apple

1 pear

1 cup of raw carrots

1 cup of chili (with or without meat)

One 4-oz turkey burger on a bun. Substitutions allowed: 4-oz veggie burger;
    4-oz cheeseburger (ground sirloin); 4 BBQ Buffalo wings; 4 oz of fish.

1 cup of green tea

2 servings of cooked veggies

2 snacks (see snacks list on page 139)

Unlimited plain water or seltzer water

EXERCISE

1 hour total:

40 minutes of cardio

20 minutes of light weights (resistance training)

NOTE: The exercise component during this module is *extremely* important.
There are more food choices you can make during these days that have a lot
more calories than other modules. If you want the choice of having those
"fun" foods, you also have to commit yourself to burning off some of those
extra calories. Please understand that not doing the recommended exercise
but indulging in the extra food could dramatically slow your weight-loss
efforts.

Day 3

2 cups of coffee (8 oz per cup). Limit sugar to 1 packet and cream or milk to 1 tsp per cup.

1 cup of cereal with ½ cup of fat-free, low-fat, reduced-fat, skim, or soy milk (see "The Scoop on Cereal," on page 117)

1 apple

1 orange (or ½ grapefruit)

1 cup of grapes

1 cup of chicken and rice (chicken can be replaced with 4–5 oz fish)

1 cup of freshly squeezed lemonade. Limit sugar to no more than 1 tsp per cup.

1 cup of vegetable soup with or without chicken; or chicken noodle soup

2 servings of cooked vegetables

2½ snacks (see snacks list on page 139)

1 cup of flavored water

Unlimited plain water

EXERCISE

45 minutes of cardio

NOTE: If you decide you want to work a little harder and add some minutes or intensity to your workout, go for it! The harder you work, the better your results and the closer you'll get to your goal. The guidelines for Day 3 on the SMOOTH module just suggest cardio, but if you add resistance training, you're ahead of the game.

Day 4

2 cups of coffee (8 oz per cup). Limit sugar to 1 packet and cream or milk to 1 tsp per cup.

1 waffle (6 inches × 6 inches) or 3 pancakes (5 inches × 5 inches) with 2 tbsp of syrup

2 pieces of fruit—your choice

1 medium-size (2 cups) green garden salad, vegetables only—no bacon bits, croutons, eggs, etc.—plus 3 tbsp of fat-free or low-fat dressing

2 cups of raw veggies (carrots, cucumber, celery, tomatoes, etc.)

1 cup of pasta with ¼ cup of tomato-based sauce (*no* creamy sauce)

2 servings of cooked vegetables

5 oz chicken, turkey, fish, or sirloin (no skin, no fried)

2 snacks (see snacks list on page 139)

1 can of diet soda or 1 cup of juice

Unlimited plain or seltzer water

EXERCISE
Rest day

Wear your pedometer and make sure you get in 10,000 steps. You are consuming more calories during this module, so it's really important on a day where you don't do your typical exercise that you at least get in the steps!

S.M.A.R.T.E.R. Choice Box

THE SCOOP ON CEREAL

Cereal is a great way to start the day, especially if you don't have a lot of time to prepare breakfast. As with any other food category, there are "good" and "bad" cereals when it comes to losing weight. Here's a list of cereals that work with the modular eating plan. Due to the enormous number of cereal brands and manufacturers, it's not possible to include every eligible cereal, but this list provides ample variety. Aim for 1 cup of cereal (unless noted) and no more than ½ cup of fat-free, skim, soy, 1% fat, or reduced-fat milk to eat with your cereal. And don't forget to eat your fruit, a great way to round off breakfast.

Cooked (measured after cooking)

    Cream of wheat

    Cream of rice

    Farina

    Grits

    Oat bran

    Oatmeal (steel-cut if possible, but instant is okay)

    Wheat hearts

Ready to eat (1 cup unless noted)

    Bran

        Wheat

        Rice bran (½ cup allowed)

        Oat bran

    Corn flakes

    Puffed corn/rice

    Shredded wheat

(continued)

S.M.A.R.T.E.R. Choice Box

Back to Nature

Granola

> Apple cinnamon (½ cup)
>
> Apple strawberry (½ cup)
>
> Cranberry pecan (½ cup)

Heart Basics

> Flax and Fiber Crunch

General Mills

> Cheerios
>
> > Original
> >
> > Apple Cinnamon
> >
> > Berry Burst, all flavors
> >
> > Frosted
> >
> > Fruity
> >
> > Honey Nut
> >
> > MultiGrain
> >
> > Oat Cluster
> >
> > Yogurt Burst, all flavors
>
> Chex
>
> > Corn
> >
> > Honey
> >
> > Multi-Bran (¾ cup)
> >
> > Rice
> >
> > Wheat (¾ cup)
>
> Cinnamon Toast Crunch
>
> Cocoa Puffs
>
> Cookie Crisps
>
> Country Corn Flakes

S.M.A.R.T.E.R. Choice Box

Fiber One

French Toast Crunch

Golden Grahams

Kix

Lucky Charms

Reese's Puffs

Total

    Whole Grain

Wheaties

Health Valley

    Amaranth Flakes

    Corn Flakes

    Crunch-Ems

    Crunchy Flakes 'n Raisins

    Crunchy Flakes 'n Strawberries

    Oat Bran Flakes

    Oat Bran Flakes with Raisins

Kashi

    7 Whole Grain

        Honey Puff

        Puffs

    Go Lean

    Heart to Heart

        Honey Toasted Oat

    Mighty Bites

        Honey Crunch

    Organic Promise

        Strawberry Fields

(continued)

S.M.A.R.T.E.R. Choice Box

Kellogg's

    All Bran

        Bran Buds

        Extra Fiber

        Original

    Corn Flakes, Original

    Corn Puffs

    Crispix, Original

    Fruit Loops, Original

        Marshmallow

    Frosted Flakes

    Fruit Harvest

    Honey Smacks

    Mini Swirlz Cinnamon Bun

    Pops, Chocolate Peanut Butter

    Product 19

    Rice Krispies

        Original

        Berry

        Frosted

        Cocoa

        Cocoa ChocoNilla

        Treats

        With Real Strawberries

    Smorz

    Special K

        Original

        Fruit & Yogurt

        Low Carb Lifestyle

        Red Berries

        Vanilla Almond

S.M.A.R.T.E.R. Choice Box

Nature's Path

        Corn flakes, all types

        Eight Grain

        Flax Plus Multigrain

        Heritage, all types

        Multigrain Oatbran Flakes

        Granola

            Ginger Zing, Hemp

            Pumpkin Flax Plus

        Kamut Crisp Flakes

New Morning

        Cocoa Crispy Rice

        Cocomotion

        Fruit-e-O's, Organic

        Oatios

            Apple Cinnamon, Organic

            Honey Almond

            Original

Post

        Alpha Bits

        Bran Flakes

        Carb Well

            Cinnamon Crunch

            Golden Crunch

        Cocoa Pebbles

        Fruity Pebbles

        Honey Bunches of Oats

        Honey Comb Strawberry Blasted

(continued)

Oreo O's with Marshmallow Bits

Waffle Crisp

Quaker

Oatmeal

Original

Instant

Oat Bran (½ cup)

Captain Crunch

Regular

Crunch Berries

Peanut Butter

Crunchy Corn Bran

Honey Graham Oh's

Life, all types

Trader Joe's

Corn flakes

Flakes n' Fruit

Frosted Flakes

High Fiber Cereal

Honey Nut O's

Joe's O's

More & Less Apple Cinnamon

Touch of Honey

Triple Berry O's

Toasted Oatmeal Flakes

The PUSH Module

Marathon runners have times in any race when they coast a little, gather their energy, and relax mentally. Then suddenly, often spontaneously, they push themselves into a sprint over a planned distance. Marathon runners pace themselves; they don't run the entire race at the same speed. The monotony of this one speed can be very taxing on the body and mind. Instead, mixing up the speed and intensity of a run over various parts of a course allows the runner to stay focused and yet relax when necessary in preparation for an aggressive push. **THE 4 DAY DIET** modular eating plan adopts a similar strategy by mixing up your food and exercise choices, allowing your body to switch gears comfortably as you consume high-octane fuel while at the same time burning excess or stored calories. The PUSH module is designed to be just that: the push of the marathon runner coming out of a steady pace to spring ahead of the pack.

The PUSH module is when everything you've learned about mental focus comes into play. Keeping yourself motivated, resisting temptation, and making every bite count will make the PUSH module easier to follow and more effective. These 4 days are just that—4 days. Don't make them any bigger than they need to be. There are 365 days in a year. Certainly it's possible for you to do almost anything for only 4 days. As always, the best way to succeed in this module is proper preparation. Remember the five P's: **P**roper **P**reparation **P**revents **P**oor **P**erformance. Get the foods you'll need and stock your fridge and cabinets accordingly.

Now take a deep breath, shake it off, stretch your arms, and then PUSSSSSSHHHHHH!!!

Day 1

2 cups of coffee (8 oz per cup). Limit sugar to 1 packet and cream or milk
   to 1 tsp per cup.

1 cup of cereal with ½ cup of fat-free, low-fat, reduced-fat, skim, or soy
   milk (see "The Scoop on Cereal," on page 117)

Grapes, unlimited

Carrots (raw or cooked), unlimited

One 4-oz serving of fish with substitutions allowed: 4 oz chicken or turkey
   or lean sirloin (no skin, no fried)

1 medium-size (2 cups) green garden salad, vegetables only—no bacon
   bits, croutons, eggs, etc.—plus 3 tbsp of fat-free or low-fat dressing

1 freshly squeezed fruit smoothie (200 calories or less; check with the
   salesperson to make sure it's less than 200 calories. Don't let them add
   any sugar.)

2 snacks (see snacks list on page 139)

2 servings of cooked veggies

Unlimited plain water

EXERCISE

2 cardio sessions of 35 minutes each

NOTE: Use your food and drinks wisely. If you eat every 2 to 3 hours, you
won't get hungry and won't feel as if you're missing something. Don't
clump your food; distribute it evenly throughout the day. Use your snacks
strategically, notably when you know that you won't be able to have the
other items because you're in transit or stuck in a meeting. Take snacks
with you so that you're prepared to keep your stomach satisfied. Before going to bed, plan and, if necessary, prepare for tomorrow.

Day 2

2 cups of coffee (8 oz per cup). Limit sugar to 1 packet and cream or milk
  to 1 tsp per cup.

2 scrambled eggs or egg whites (optional: add ¼ cup of chopped vegetables; 1
  tsp of oil for cooking)

1 slice of bacon

1 cup of mixed fruit

1 cup of green tea or other types

1 cup of cooked lentils

1 medium-size (2 cups) green garden salad, vegetables only—no bacon bits,
  croutons, eggs, etc.—plus 3 tbsp of fat-free or low-fat dressing

1 apple

Sliced cucumbers unlimited (dip in fat-free dressing, if desired)

5 oz of fish. Substitutions allowed: 5 oz skinless chicken or turkey (not
  fried) or sirloin steak or ground sirloin.

2 cups of flavored water, regular water, or seltzer water

Unlimited plain water

EXERCISE

1 hour of cardio—you can do it all at once or divide into two sessions

8,000 steps using your pedometer to count. Don't wear the pedometer
  while exercising.

Day 3

2 cups of coffee (8 oz per cup). Limit sugar to 1 packet and cream or milk
   to 1 tsp per cup.

1 apple

1 pear

1 orange

1 cup of cooked beans, chickpeas, lentils, or other legumes (but *no* baked
   beans)

1 medium-size (2 cups) green garden salad, vegetables only—no bacon bits,
   croutons, eggs, etc.—plus 3 tbsp of fat-free or low-fat dressing

2 cups of raw or cooked carrots

2 snacks (see snacks list on page 139)

1 cup of freshly squeezed lemonade. Limit sugar to no more than 1 tsp per
   cup.

5 oz of skinless turkey or chicken (no skin, no fried)

2 servings of cooked vegetables

Unlimited plain water

EXERCISE

Rest day

Walk 10,000 steps using your pedometer to count.

Day 4

2 cups coffee (8 oz per cup). Limit sugar to 1 packet and cream or milk to 1 tsp per cup.

1 egg, scrambled (1 tsp of oil for cooking allowed)

1 apple

1 pear

1 cup of cooked beans, chickpeas, lentils or other legumes (but no baked beans)

2 medium-size (2 cups) green garden salads, vegetables only—no bacon bits, croutons, eggs, etc.—plus 3 tbsp of fat-free or low-fat dressing and unlimited grapes

1 cup of carrots

1 small fresh-fruit cup

Unlimited cucumbers (optional: 3 tbsp of fat-free or low-fat dressing)

5 oz of fish

Unlimited plain water

EXERCISE

60 minutes of cardio (if necessary, break it up)

The PACE Module

The biggest mistake an inexperienced marathon runner can make is to run on emotion rather than on strategy. The best chance a runner has to complete the race and record the best possible time is through planned pacing. Marathon strategists universally agree that pacing is critical throughout the entire race and that violating it can lead to negative results, even injury. Watch the beginning of a marathon with enthusiastic runners sprinting out to the front of the pack, feeling great about themselves, caught up in the moment and running on adrenaline. Some believe they can run hard during the first half of the race and build up a reserve so that they can coast in the second half. This is a fallacy and a tactic that almost always ends in failure or injury. The same can be said of any weight-loss journey. Sprinting too hard early and not pacing yourself can be the biggest mistake you make.

Similar to the marathon course, where the topography of the land is constantly changing, so is the path of your weight-loss journey. The terrain is hilly at times, smooth at others, and uneven in some spots. You have to pace yourself throughout the entire journey so that you don't twist an ankle on a slippery turn or run out of steam before you reach the finish line. The PACE module is designed to keep you moving forward but at a speed that will encourage you to finish strong during the later stages of the race. Keep this in mind as you PACE yourself over the next four days. Enjoy!

Day 1

2 cups of coffee (8 oz per cup). Limit sugar to 1 packet and cream or milk to 1 tsp per cup.

1 cup of cereal (see "The Scoop on Cereal," on page 117)

One 6-oz low-fat or fat-free yogurt *without* "fruit on the bottom." Add your own fresh fruit if you like.

4 oz of fish, skinless chicken, or turkey, not fried, or lean sirloin

1 medium-size (2 cups) green garden salad, vegetables only—no bacon bits, croutons, eggs, etc.—plus 3 tbsp of fat-free or low-fat dressing

2 servings of vegetables

1 cup of cooked brown rice

1 cup of cooked beans, chickpeas, lentils, or other legumes (but no baked beans)

2 snacks (see snacks list on page 139)

1 cup of flavored water

Unlimited plain water

EXERCISE

30 minutes of cardio (if necessary, break it up)

20 minutes of light weights (resistance training)

Day 2

2 cups of coffee (8 oz per cup). Limit sugar to 1 packet and cream or milk
   to 1 tsp per cup.

1 egg white omelet with vegetables (2 egg whites or ½ cup of egg beaters or
   1 whole egg plus ¼ cup of chopped vegetables; 1 tsp of oil for cooking)

3 pieces of fruit

1 sandwich: 3 ounces of turkey, chicken, or ham on 2 slices of whole-grain or
   whole wheat bread (½ teaspoon of mayonnaise or 1 teaspoon of mustard
   allowed; you can also add lettuce and sliced tomatoes)

1 cup of freshly squeezed juice

1 large-size (3 cups) green garden salad, vegetables only—no bacon bits,
   croutons, eggs, etc.—plus 3 tbsp of fat-free or low-fat dressing

½ cup of cooked beans, chickpeas, lentils, or other legumes (but no baked
   beans)

5-oz veggie burger. Substitutions allowed: 5-oz turkey burger; 5-oz cheeseburger (ground sirloin); 4 BBQ buffalo wings; 5 oz of fish.

2 snacks (see snacks list on page 139)

Unlimited plain water or seltzer water

1 can of diet soda

EXERCISE

45 minutes of cardio (if necessary, break it up)

Day 3

2 cups of coffee (8 oz per cup). Limit sugar to 1 packet and cream or milk to 1 tsp per cup.

Two 3-inch pancakes or two 3-inch waffles. Use no more than 1 tbsp of syrup.

2 pieces of fruit

1 cup of green tea or other types of tea

1 medium-size (2 cups) green garden salad, vegetables only—no bacon bits, croutons, eggs, etc.—plus 3 tbsp of fat-free or low-fat dressing

1 cup of vegetable soup (with or without chicken) or chicken noodle soup

2 servings of cooked vegetables

5 oz of fish (substitutions allowed: 5 oz of skinless chicken or turkey, not fried, or sirloin steak or ground sirloin)

One 8-oz diet soda

Unlimited plain water

EXERCISE

30 minutes of cardio

20 minutes of resistance training

Day 4

2 cups of coffee (8 oz per cup). Limit sugar to 1 packet and cream or milk to 1 tsp per cup.

One 6-oz low-fat or fat-free yogurt *without* "fruit on the bottom." Add your own fresh fruit if you like.

1 sandwich: 3 oz of turkey, chicken, or ham on 2 slices of whole-grain or whole wheat bread, with ½ tsp of mayonnaise or 1 tsp of mustard allowed. You can also add lettuce and sliced tomatoes.

2 servings of fruit

1 cup of cooked brown rice (measured after cooking)

1 small-size (1 cup) green garden salad, vegetables only—no bacon bits, croutons, eggs, etc.—plus 3 tbsp of fat-free or low-fat dressing

1 cup of chili (with or without meat)

2 servings of cooked vegetables

1 cup of flavored water

Unlimited plain water

EXERCISE

Rest day

Walk 10,000 steps using your pedometer to count.

The VIGOROUS Module

You are approaching the finish line. Think of yourself as a runner who has about 3 minutes left in the race. If you've followed your strategy up to this point, it will pay off. While others might be exhausted and barely able to stand on their two feet, you won't just run across the finish line, you'll *sprint*. This is the "kick" portion of the race where you go really hard for a short period of time and throw your hands up in victory as you break through the tape. You've seen the image many times, the end of a grueling race—almost 25 miles, and somehow, in some way, those runners are able to kick into high gear and duel the last several hundred yards. Well, now it's your turn.

The VIGOROUS module is designed to challenge you, but with all that you've learned, it's a challenge that you are well prepared to meet head-on and win. Summoning your mental strength to get through these three days is as critical as preparation. Make sure you have the food and drink the VIGOROUS module calls for in your house or at least access to them if that means ordering in from a local restaurant. Don't look at the next four days as a chore but as a final lap to a great victory that you can repeat as often as you like.

Finishing VIGOROUS doesn't mean you've necessarily reached your ultimate goal. You may well have more road to cover on your journey, and that's completely fine. You can go back and do the modules again from the beginning or even switch the order. Just remember that each module has a purpose, and when following that module for the second time, the original purpose should be maintained.

Day 1

2 cups of coffee (8 oz per cup). Limit sugar to 1 packet and cream or milk to 1 tsp per cup.

One 6-oz low-fat or fat-free yogurt *without* "fruit on the bottom." Add your own fresh fruit if you like.

2 cups of carrots (raw or cooked)

2 cups of grapes

1 cup of soup (non-creamy)

1 medium-size (2 cups) green garden salad, vegetables only—no bacon bits, croutons, eggs, etc.—plus 3 tbsp of fat-free or low-fat dressing

1 freshly squeezed fruit smoothie—200 calories or less. Check with the salesperson to be sure it's less than 200 calories. No sugar should be added.

5 oz of fish. Substitutions allowed: 5 oz of skinless chicken or turkey (not fried) or sirloin steak or lean sirloin.

2 servings of cooked vegetables

Unlimited water

EXERCISE

40 minutes of cardio (if necessary, break it up)

Day 2

One 6-oz low-fat or fat-free yogurt *without* "fruit on the bottom." Add your own fresh fruit if you like.

1 apple

1 pear

1 banana

½ large cucumber, sliced, with 2 tbsp of fat-free or low-fat dressing

1 large-size (3 cups) green garden salad, vegetables only—no bacon bits, no croutons, no eggs, etc.—plus 3 tbsp of fat-free or low-fat dressing

One 8-oz cup of flavored water. You might want to keep it nice and chilled and drink it throughout the day.

1½ cups of soup (non-creamy)

2 servings of cooked vegetables

2 snacks (see snacks list on page 139)

Unlimited plain water

EXERCISE

50 minutes of cardio (if necessary, break it up)

Day 3

2 cups of coffee (8 oz per cup). Limit sugar to 1 packet and cream or milk
   to 1 tsp per cup.
1 egg white omelet with vegetables (2 egg whites or ½ cup of Egg Beaters or
   1 whole egg plus ¼ cup of chopped vegetables)
2 servings of fruit
1 medium-size (2 cups) green garden salad, vegetables only—no bacon bits,
   croutons, eggs, etc.—plus 3 tbsp of fat-free or low-fat dressing
5 oz of fish. Substitutions allowed: 5 oz of chicken or turkey or lean sirloin
   (no skin, no fried).
1 cup of green tea or other type of tea
2 servings of cooked vegetables
2 snacks (see snacks list on page 139)
Unlimited plain water

EXERCISE
Rest day

Day 4

One 6-oz low-fat or fat-free yogurt *without* "fruit on the bottom." Add fresh fruit instead.

2 cups of coffee (8 oz per cup). Limit sugar to 1 packet and cream or milk to 1 tsp per cup.

2 cups of grapes

2 cups of raw baby carrots

1½ cup of soup (non-creamy)

1 large-size (3 cups) green garden salad with strips of chicken (3 oz)—no bacon bits, croutons, eggs, etc.—plus 3 tbsp of fat-free or low-fat dressing

1 freshly squeezed fruit smoothie—200 calories or less. Check with the salesperson to be sure it's less than 200 calories. No sugar should be added.

5 oz of skinless chicken or turkey, not fried, or lean sirloin, substitute with fish if preferred

2 servings of cooked vegetables

Unlimited plain or seltzer water

EXERCISE

50 minutes of cardio (if necessary, break it up)

CHAPTER 9

Healthy, Low-Calorie Snacks (150 calories or less per snack)

20 raw almonds

½ apple, sliced, with 2 teaspoons peanut butter

2 cups air-popped popcorn (without butter or other condiments)

1 cup sliced bananas with fresh raspberries

4 mini rice cakes with 2 tablespoons low-fat cottage cheese

½ cup edamame (frozen soybeans)

1 cup grapes

1 large dill pickle wrapped in 1 thin slice Swiss cheese

½ small avocado

1 fat-free chocolate pudding cup

6 ounces fat-free plain yogurt topped with ⅓ cup raspberries

½ cup low-fat cottage cheese with 5 strawberries

2 large graham cracker squares with 1 teaspoon peanut butter

½ cup sugar-free Jell-O and 2 tablespoons reduced-fat whipped topping

¼ cup fat-free ranch dressing with a cup of mixed raw veggies

1 large orange, sliced

1 slice of raisin bread

6 ounces tossed salad with lettuce, tomato, 1 tablespoon low-fat shredded cheese, cucumber, and ¼ cup fat-free dressing (but no bacon bits or croutons)

½ cup frozen low-fat yogurt topped with ½ cup blueberries, strawberries, or raspberries

4 ounces water-packed tuna

1–2 cups cherry tomatoes

4 ounces cooked whole-grain noodles with 1 small fresh tomato and ½ ounce hard cheese

⅓ cup unsweetened applesauce with 1 slice whole-wheat toast

1 cup baby carrots

3 ounces lean roast beef

1 medium banana and 1 tablespoon cottage cheese

1 Yoplait Light Smoothie

1 seven-grain Belgian waffle, 1 teaspoon syrup allowed

60 Pepperidge Farm Baby Goldfish Crackers

½ medium cantaloupe

2 stalks celery and 2 ounces hummus

Four large (1 ounce) marshmallows

8 Wheat Thins crackers with 2 teaspoons peanut butter

1 cup tomato soup made with water

½ whole-grain bagel with 1½ teaspoons light cream cheese

½ cup frozen orange juice (eat it like an Italian ice or sorbet)

1 Fudgsicle

¾ cup unsweetened applesauce with ¼ teaspoon cinnamon

1 small baked sweet potato with 2 tablespoons fat-free sour cream

3 Quaker Cheddar Cheese Rice Cakes

Half a "finger" of string cheese with 5 whole wheat crackers

½ cup peaches with ½ cup cottage cheese

MorningStar Farms cheddar burger on whole wheat bun with 1 teaspoon ketchup or mustard

½ cup fat-free and sugar-free instant or packaged pudding

1 cup fresh strawberries

½ cup fresh blueberries

½ cup vegetable soup

15 Back to Nature Sesame Ginger Rice Thins

3 domino-size slices low-fat cheese

5 slices Melba toast

4 rye crispbread crackers

8 saltine crackers with 2 teaspoons peanut butter (my personal favorite!)

Half a turkey sandwich on whole-grain, seven-grain, or multigrain bread with 1 teaspoon mustard or low-fat mayonnaise

4 small ginger snaps

½ cup bran cereal with ¼ cup blueberries

2 tablespoons sunflower seeds

CHAPTER 10

Recipes

I'm excited to present the following recipes. Big City Chefs worked hard to provide tasty recipes that you can prepare right at home. These recipes are only meant to be suggestions for some of the different dishes you can prepare as you go through the modules of **THE 4 DAY DIET**. By no means are these recipes meant to be a comprehensive list, and you can use other healthy recipes as long as they follow the guidelines of the diet.

You will find that most of these recipes are easy to follow, and the ingredients can be found at any decent grocery store. You will be able to prepare most of them in under one hour. Some recipes are more ambitious, however. They require a few more ingredients, will take a little longer to cook, and are a little more challenging to prepare. I include these recipes because many of you have asked for menu items that would test your cooking skills a little more.

Cooking should be fun, and part of the fun is finding new and interesting ingredients, making tasty combinations you never thought you'd find appealing, and, whenever possible, cooking along with others in your household. The closer you get to fresh ingredients and to really knowing what goes into what you eat, the more you'll enjoy your meals, the more satisfied you'll be, and the more **THE 4 DAY DIET** will work for you. If you need to make substitutions for medical reasons or because you simply can't find the ingredients listed, go ahead and do so, but just keep in mind the rules of the diet.

Make your **4 DAY DIET** meals an adventure. Switch where you shop; visit the farmer's market, ethnic food stores, or even an unfamiliar supermarket in a new neighborhood to freshen the way you look at ingredients and cooking.

Enjoy these recipes, and I hope this will finally prove that being on a diet doesn't mean you can't have tasty and interesting food at every meal.

Bon appétit!

Breakfast

· WHOLE WHEAT PANCAKES WITH LOW-CALORIE ·
SYRUP AND FRESH BERRIES

SERVES 4

Serve pancakes with a drizzle of low-calorie syrup and fresh berries.

2 cups whole wheat flour

1 teaspoon canola oil

1 tablespoon honey

1 tablespoon baking powder

2 eggs

2 cups skim milk

¼ cup low-calorie pancake syrup

1 cup assorted berries, such as
   strawberries and blueberries

Combine flour, oil, honey, baking powder, eggs, and milk in a large bowl.
   Whisk until smooth.

Spray a griddle or nonstick pan with nonstick cooking spray. Heat to medium
   heat and pour batter onto it by ¼ cupfuls.

When bubbles appear and burst on top, flip the pancakes and cook until
   springy to the touch.

PER SERVING (EXCLUDING UNKNOWN ITEMS): 347 calories; 5 g fat (12.5% calories from
fat); 16 g protein; 64 g carbohydrate; 8 g dietary fiber; 108 mg cholesterol; 497 mg
sodium.

• FRESH FRUIT AND BRAN BREAKFAST SMOOTHIE •

SERVES 4

This breakfast can be made in minutes and is great on the go.

4 ripe bananas or peaches or
    nectarines, peeled and
    roughly chopped

2 cups nonfat yogurt
4 teaspoons honey
4 tablespoons natural bran

Combine the fruit, yogurt, honey, and bran in a blender or food processor. Whirl until smooth. Pour into a tall glass.

PER SERVING (EXCLUDING UNKNOWN ITEMS): 201 calories; 1 g fat (3.7% calories from fat); 8 g protein; 45 g carbohydrate; 4 g dietary fiber; 2 mg cholesterol; 88 mg sodium.

· STEEL-CUT OATMEAL WITH APPLES, ·
ALMONDS, AND DATES

SERVES 4

3 cups water

1 teaspoon ground cinnamon

¼ teaspoon kosher salt

1¼ cups steel-cut oats

1 small apple, chopped

2 tablespoons sliced almonds

¼ cup pitted dates, chopped

1 tablespoon brown sugar

3 cups skim milk

In a medium saucepan, combine the water, cinnamon, and salt. Bring to a boil, then stir in the oats. Cook for 20 minutes, stirring occasionally. After the first 15 minutes, add the chopped apple and allow to cook slightly. Let the oatmeal mixture stand, covered, until desired consistency. Divide the oatmeal among serving bowls and top with almonds, dates, brown sugar, and milk.

PER SERVING (EXCLUDING UNKNOWN ITEMS): 268 calories; 5 g fat (15.6% calories from fat); 12 g protein; 46 g carbohydrate; 6 g dietary fiber; 3 mg cholesterol; 220 mg sodium.

· YOGURT WITH GRANOLA, MANGOES, · AND CRYSTALLIZED GINGER

SERVES 4

This makes a very quick on the go breakfast. Be sure to look for granola with whole oats and grains and no added sugar, or make your own. For a health bonus, choose yogurt with active cultures.

2 tablespoons chopped
    crystallized ginger
8 ounces granola
2 cups nonfat yogurt

2 ripe mangoes, peeled, pitted,
    and diced
Ground cinnamon (optional)

Toss the chopped crystallized ginger with the granola. In a small bowl or a tall to-go cup (for transport), layer the yogurt, granola-ginger mixture, and mangoes in alternating layers. Sprinkle with cinnamon if desired.

PER SERVING (EXCLUDING UNKNOWN ITEMS): 357 calories; 16 g fat (37.7% calories from fat); 13 g protein; 45 g carbohydrate; 6 g dietary fiber; 2 mg cholesterol; 96 mg sodium.

· APPLE AND ALMOND WHOLE WHEAT PANCAKES ·

SERVES 4

½ cup whole wheat flour
½ cup unbleached flour
1 tablespoon brown sugar
1½ teaspoons baking powder
¼ teaspoon salt

2 eggs, separated
4 tablespoons canola oil
½ cup buttermilk
½ cup fresh, unfiltered apple juice
¼ cup chopped almonds

In a mixing bowl, combine the flours, sugar, baking powder, and salt.

Beat the egg yolks with the oil, buttermilk, and apple juice. Stir into the flour mixture with nuts just until all ingredients are moistened. Beat the egg whites until stiff and fold into the batter.

Spoon the batter onto a hot griddle that has been coated with nonstick cooking spray, and turn once when bubbles appear. Makes 8 to 10 pancakes.

PER SERVING (EXCLUDING UNKNOWN ITEMS): 348 calories; 21 g fat (54% calories from fat); 10 g protein; 31 g carbohydrate; 2 g dietary fiber; 107 mg cholesterol; 371 mg sodium.

ASIAN BREAKFAST STIR-FRY WITH SOBA NOODLES AND FRESH VEGETABLES

SERVES 4

2 teaspoons canola oil

4 large eggs

2 tablespoons slivered ginger

2 scallions, thinly sliced

1 cup soba noodles, cooked

12 snow peas

8 baby corn

2 tomatoes, sliced

2 tablespoons soy sauce

2 tablespoons cilantro leaves, minced

Add ½ teaspoon oil to a sauté pan over medium heat. Add the eggs and cook
into a thin omelet. Remove from heat and slice into strips.

Add the remaining oil to the pan. Add the ginger, green onions, snow peas,
and baby corn. Cook over medium heat until the ginger is fragrant and
snow peas turn bright green, about 1 minute, then add the noodles. Sauté
until warm, stirring constantly.

Add the egg strips, tomatoes, and soy sauce. Stir over medium heat until hot.
Sprinkle each serving with 1 tablespoon chopped cilantro.

PER SERVING (EXCLUDING UNKNOWN ITEMS): 337 calories; 8 g fat (21.5% calories from
fat); 23 g protein; 44 g carbohydrate; 7 g dietary fiber; 212 mg cholesterol; 746 mg
sodium.

• BREAKFAST BURRITO WITH SCRAMBLED EGG • WHITES, PINTO BEANS, SALSA, AND TURKEY SAUSAGE

SERVES 4

½ cup canned pinto beans, rinsed
   and drained
1 teaspoon canola oil
8 ounces turkey breakfast sausage,
   crumbled

8 egg whites
Salt and pepper to taste
2 whole wheat tortillas
1 cup salsa

Heat the pinto beans in the microwave until hot, then mash them lightly with a fork. In a nonstick skillet over medium heat, heat half the oil and add the turkey sausage until fully cooked.

Beat the egg whites in a small bowl and season with salt and pepper to taste. Heat the remaining oil in a small nonstick skillet over medium heat and cook the egg whites until set.

Soften the tortillas by warming them between two damp paper towels for ten seconds in the microwave. Divide pinto bean mash along the center of each tortilla, top with half the egg whites and sausage, top that with the salsa, and fold up. Cut burritos in half; each half is one serving.

PER SERVING (EXCLUDING UNKNOWN ITEMS): 349 calories; 14 g fat (35.2% calories from fat); 23 g protein; 34 g carbohydrate; 8 g dietary fiber; 45 mg cholesterol; 964 mg sodium.

· SWEET POTATO LATKES WITH APPLE SAUCE ·

SERVES 4

4 medium sweet potatoes

1 medium yellow onion

1 egg

⅓ cup flour

1 teaspoon kosher salt

1 cup unsweetened applesauce

Peel and grate the sweet potatoes into a mixing bowl and squeeze out any liquid. Peel and grate the onion into the sweet potatoes. Add the egg, flour, and salt. Stir to make a smooth batter that will drop heavily from the spoon to form a large pancake. Let the batter rest for 15 minutes.

Bake the pancakes in a shallow baking pan for 45 minutes at 350°F until nicely browned. Cut into squares and serve hot. They may also be baked individually in a small muffin pan that has been coated with nonstick cooking spray.

Serve warm with fresh applesauce.

Note: Substitute brown rice flour for the regular flour to make these pancakes light and crisp.

PER SERVING (EXCLUDING UNKNOWN ITEMS): 239 calories; 2 g fat (7.7% calories from fat); 5 g protein; 51 g carbohydrate; 6 g dietary fiber; 53 mg cholesterol; 507 mg sodium.

CALIFORNIA OMELET WITH EGG WHITES, • ARTICHOKES, AVOCADO, AND JACK CHEESE

SERVES 4

12 egg whites

2 tablespoons skim milk

Salt and pepper to taste

8 frozen artichoke hearts, thawed and diced

1 cup fresh tomato salsa

1 cup reduced-fat Monterey Jack cheese

½ avocado, diced

Whisk the eggs whites, milk, salt, and pepper together. In a medium nonstick skillet coated with nonstick spray, cook the eggs over medium heat until just set. Add the artichoke hearts, salsa, and cheese to one side of the omelet. Fold the other half of the omelet over the filling. Top with diced avocado and serve.

PER SERVING (EXCLUDING UNKNOWN ITEMS): 265 calories; 7 g fat (23.6% calories from fat); 26 g protein; 27 g carbohydrate; 11 g dietary fiber; 10 mg cholesterol; 763 mg sodium.

• COUNTRY BREAKFAST TURKEY PATTY WITH •
OATMEAL AND SIDE OF FRUIT

SERVES 4

8 ounces ground turkey

2 eggs

2 tablespoons chopped red bell
  pepper

2 tablespoons diced yellow onion

1 teaspoon fresh thyme

Salt and pepper to taste

1 tablespoon olive oil

½ cup dry instant oats

1 cup skim milk

1 cup sliced strawberries

Combine the ground turkey, eggs, bell pepper, onion, thyme, salt, and
pepper. Form into 4 patties. Sauté the patties in olive oil until cooked
through and golden brown on both sides, approximately 3 minutes on each
side depending on their thickness.

Cook the oats in milk according to the package instructions.

Serve each patty with a side of sliced strawberries and oatmeal.

PER SERVING (EXCLUDING UNKNOWN ITEMS): 224 calories; 11 g fat (46.1% calories
from fat); 17 g protein; 13 g carbohydrate; 2 g dietary fiber; 152 mg cholesterol; 223 mg
sodium.

CURRIED EGGS BENEDICT WITH WHOLE WHEAT • ENGLISH MUFFINS

SERVES 4

1 cup finely chopped onion

1 tablespoon canola oil

2 tablespoons curry powder

1 tablespoon whole wheat flour

¾ cup skim milk

4 whole wheat English muffins

1 large tomato, sliced

8 poached eggs

Chopped fresh cilantro or parsley

Sauté the onion in the canola oil until soft. Stir in the curry and flour and heat for 2 minutes. Slowly add the milk, stirring constantly as the sauce thickens.

Split and toast the muffins and top each half with a tomato slice, a poached egg, and curry sauce. Garnish with cilantro or parsley and serve.

PER SERVING (EXCLUDING UNKNOWN ITEMS): 367 calories; 15 g fat (37% calories from fat); 21 g protein; 38 g carbohydrate; 6 g dietary fiber; 424 mg cholesterol; 760 mg sodium.

· EGG WHITE AND TURKEY BACON BREAKFAST · BURRITO WITH PINEAPPLE SALSA

SERVES 4

This is a great breakfast choice for the PROTEIN STRETCH module—it would also make a great lunch or dinner!

8 slices turkey bacon

¼ cup chopped green pepper

¼ cup sliced yellow onion

8 egg whites, beaten

⅛ teaspoon freshly ground
   black pepper

½ cup grated reduced-fat cheddar cheese

4 whole wheat tortillas

½ cup fresh tomato salsa

½ cup chopped fresh pineapple

Vegetable spray

Microwave the bacon, arranging 4 slices on a paper plate and covering with a paper towel. Arrange the remaining 4 slices on top of the towel and cover with another paper towel. Microwave on high power for 7 to 8 minutes, until the bacon is crisp. Crumble and set aside.

Coat a large nonstick skillet with vegetable spray and cook the green pepper and onion over medium-high heat for 3 to 4 minutes, until the vegetables are tender.

Lower the heat to medium and add the egg whites and pepper to the vegetables. Cook for 2 to 3 minutes, until the eggs are almost done.

Remove the skillet from the heat and stir in the cheese and bacon.

Wrap the tortillas in a paper towel and microwave on high for 5 to 20 seconds to soften them. Meanwhile, combine the tomato salsa with the pineapple.

Place ¼ cup of the mixture on the lower third of each tortilla. Roll up the tortilla, top with salsa, and serve.

PER SERVING (EXCLUDING UNKNOWN ITEMS): 291 calories; 9 g fat (27.9% calories from fat); 19 g protein; 33 g carbohydrate; 3 g dietary fiber; 28 mg cholesterol; 1086 mg sodium.

Note: Fat-free tortillas can be substituted for wheat tortillas.

• EGG WHITE OMELET WITH BASIL PESTO • AND FRESH FRUIT

SERVES 4

1 cup basil leaves
1 tomato, chopped
2 cloves garlic, peeled and minced
1 tablespoon pine nuts (pignoli,
   toasted recommended but you
   can try others)

Salt to taste
18 egg whites
Pepper to taste
2 tablespoons olive oil
1 cup fresh fruit

To make the pesto: Rinse and drain the basil leaves. In a blender or food processor, combine the basil, tomato, garlic, pine nuts, and 1¼ teaspoons salt. Puree until smooth. Make sure you get all the ingredients at the side of the processor into the blend.

To make each omelet: Whisk together the egg whites, salt, and pepper. In a nonstick omelet pan, heat one-fourth of the oil and pour in one-fourth of the egg white mixture. Cook until just set, stirring constantly with a rubber spatula. Fold over, drizzle with one-fourth of the pesto, and serve with ¼ cup fresh fruit.

PER SERVING (EXCLUDING UNKNOWN ITEMS): 160 calories; 8 g fat (45.6% calories from fat); 17 g protein; 5 g carbohydrate; 1 g dietary fiber; 0 mg cholesterol; 815 mg sodium.

· HOMEMADE MUESLI AND YOGURT PARFAIT ·

SERVES 8

This is a great quick on-the-go breakfast. You may also store larger quantities of muesli in an airtight container.

8 ounces rolled oats

8 ounces barley flakes

2 ounces mixed dry-roasted nuts, chopped

2 ounces dried fruit, chopped

12 ounces nonfat yogurt

Stir together all the dry ingredients until evenly mixed.

In a tall glass, layer alternating layers of muesli and yogurt.

PER SERVING (EXCLUDING UNKNOWN ITEMS): 301 calories; 7 g fat (21.4% calories from fat); 13 g protein; 48 g carbohydrate; 7 g dietary fiber; 1 mg cholesterol; 37 mg sodium.

· LOW-CALORIE WESTERN OMELET WITH TURKEY · HAM AND BELL PEPPERS

SERVES 4

1 teaspoon canola oil

1 medium red bell pepper, cored, seeded, and cut into strips

1 medium green bell pepper, cored, seeded, and cut into strips

4 ounces turkey ham, cut into strips (about 1 cup)

Salt and pepper to taste

4 large eggs

4 large egg whites

4 tablespoons minced fresh parsley (optional)

Heat the canola oil in a 10-inch nonstick skillet over medium-high heat. Add the peppers and turkey ham. Cook for a few minutes, stirring frequently, until the peppers are crisp-tender. Season lightly with salt and pepper. Remove from the heat but keep warm.

In a small bowl using a wire whisk or fork, beat 1 egg and 1 egg white until blended and frothy. Spray a 6-inch nonstick skillet or omelet pan with nonstick vegetable spray. Set over medium heat. Pour the egg mixture into the skillet. Using the flat side of a fork, stir briskly in a circular motion while shaking the pan back and forth over the heat. When the liquid has just begun to set, stop stirring. Let the omelet cook for 30 to 40 seconds more, until the edges and bottom are set but the center is still soft. Loosen the omelet around the edges with a spatula until it moves freely. Remove from the heat.

Arrange one-fourth of the reserved pepper mixture on the side of the omelet farthest away from the skillet handle. Tilt the handle up. Using the spatula, lift the edge of the omelet nearest the handle up and over the peppers. Slide the omelet onto a plate. Garnish with parsley if desired. Serve immediately. Repeat to make additional omelets.

PER SERVING (EXCLUDING UNKNOWN ITEMS): 154 calories; 8 g fat (45.5% calories from fat); 16 g protein; 5 g carbohydrate; 1 g dietary fiber; 228 mg cholesterol; 410 mg sodium.

• NUTTY OATMEAL AND WHOLE WHEAT •
BREAKFAST BREAD PUDDING

SERVES 4

4 cups whole wheat bread cubes,
  lightly toasted
½ cup steel-cut oatmeal (or instant
  oatmeal)
3 large eggs, lightly beaten
⅓ cup skim milk

2 tablespoons brown sugar
2 teaspoons vanilla extract
2 teaspoons nutmeg
½ cup dried fruit
¼ cup slivered almonds

Fill a 9-by-14-inch oven-safe bowl one-half to two-thirds full with the bread
  cubes. Add the oatmeal. In a separate bowl, beat the eggs, milk, sugar,
  vanilla, and nutmeg, and pour over the bread and oatmeal. Add the dried
  fruit and stir to combine. Bake until the pudding has risen high and turned
  medium brown (45 to 60 minutes). It will rise like a soufflé and fall as it
  cools. Sprinkle with almonds.
Serve warm smothered with skim milk for a perfect cold weather breakfast.

PER SERVING (EXCLUDING UNKNOWN ITEMS): 334 calories; 11 g fat (30.3% calories
from fat); 13 g protein; 45 g carbohydrate; 4 g dietary fiber; 159 mg cholesterol; 327 mg
sodium.

• MUSHROOM FRITTATA WITH SPICY TOMATO RELISH •

SERVES 4

You can use any combination of your favorite mushrooms for this very low-calorie recipe, which is delicious served hot or cold.

Tomato Relish:

2 ripe tomatoes

2 tablespoons finely diced yellow onion

1 tablespoon minced fresh parsley

1 teaspoon red pepper flakes

¼ cup red wine vinegar

Salt and pepper to taste

Mushroom Frittata:

2 tablespoons extra-virgin olive oil

1 cup sliced fresh mushrooms

4 cloves garlic, peeled and minced

5 eggs, lightly beaten

5 egg whites, lightly beaten

2 tablespoons minced fresh herbs

To make the relish: Combine the tomatoes, onion, parsley, red pepper flakes, vinegar, salt, and pepper in a bowl and blend well. Set aside at room temperature while making the frittata.

To make the frittata: Heat half of the oil in a 12-inch nonstick skillet over medium heat. Add the mushrooms and cook until tender, about 4 minutes. Add the garlic and cook, stirring, for 30 seconds. Transfer to a plate and keep warm. Wipe out the skillet.

Whisk the eggs and egg whites together with the fresh herbs in a medium bowl. Stir in salt, pepper, and the mushroom-garlic mixture. In the meantime, preheat a broiler and set an oven rack about 4 inches from the top. Brush the skillet with the remaining oil and place over medium heat. Pour in the egg mixture and tilt to distribute evenly. Reduce the heat to medium-low and cook until the bottom is light golden. Lift the edges of the egg mixture to allow uncooked egg to flow underneath, 3 to 4 minutes. Place the pan under the broiler and cook until the top is set, 1½ to 2½ minutes. Slide the frittata onto a platter and cut into wedges, topped with a spoonful of tomato relish.

PER SERVING (EXCLUDING UNKNOWN ITEMS): 201 calories; 13 g fat (58.9% calories from fat); 14 g protein; 7 g carbohydrate; 1 g dietary fiber; 265 mg cholesterol; 167 mg sodium.

OAT BRAN AND APPLE CEREAL WITH MAPLE SYRUP AND RAISINS

SERVES 4

4 cups water

1⅓ cups oat bran

½ cup seedless raisins

1 apple, grated

1 tablespoon maple syrup

½ teaspoon ground caraway seeds (optional)

½ teaspoon ground cinnamon

1 cup skim milk

In a 2-quart saucepan, bring the water and oat bran to a vigorous boil, stirring frequently. Reduce the heat to low and cook for 2 minutes, stirring frequently, until thick. Remove from the heat and stir in the raisins, apple, maple syrup, caraway seeds (if using), and cinnamon. Let stand for 5 minutes. Spoon into bowls and serve with the milk.

PER SERVING (EXCLUDING UNKNOWN ITEMS): 188 calories; 3 g fat (9.5% calories from fat); 8 g protein; 47 g carbohydrate; 7 g dietary fiber; 1 mg cholesterol; 43 mg sodium.

· POACHED EGG WITH TURKEY BACON, GRILLED · TOMATO, AND BLACK BEANS

SERVES 4

8 turkey bacon slices

2 tomatoes, halved

12 ounces canned black beans,
   rinsed and drained

Salt and pepper to taste

8 eggs

In a nonstick skillet over medium-low heat, slowly heat the turkey bacon until crisp. Meanwhile, heat a heavy cast-iron grill pan or indoor grill over medium-high heat. Place 4 tomato halves, cut side down, on the grill and cook until the bottoms have nice grill marks and soften slightly, about 2 minutes. Turn over and cook another 2 minutes, until the tomatoes are warm but not hot throughout. Set aside.

Heat the black beans in a microwave until hot and then mash lightly with a fork. Season with salt and pepper.

Place 2 inches of water in a pan that is at least 3 inches deep. Heat the water to a boil, then lower it to a simmer and allow it to cool for a few minutes. Working with the eggs one at a time, crack each egg into a saucer or small cup, then carefully slide it into the simmering water right at the surface. Turn off the stove and set a timer for 3 minutes for a medium-cooked egg. Remove the egg from the water with a slotted spoon.

To serve, make two pools of black bean mash on each plate. Top each with a grilled tomato half, one slice of bacon, and a poached egg, for two eggs per serving.

PER SERVING (EXCLUDING UNKNOWN ITEMS): 301 calories; 16 g fat (49.5% calories from fat); 22 g protein; 15 g carbohydrate; 5 g dietary fiber; 449 mg cholesterol; 776 mg sodium.

• SOUTHWESTERN BAKED EGGS •

SERVES 4

1 tablespoon unsalted butter
8 large eggs
6 tablespoons skim milk
¾ teaspoon salt
¼ teaspoon ground black pepper

⅔ cup shredded low-fat cheddar cheese
4 ounces diced green chilies, seeded and
  chopped
Chili, ketchup, or tomato sauce (optional)
1 sliced tomato

Put butter in 8-inch square baking pan. Set in 350°F oven to melt. Shake the
  pan to distribute the butter evenly.

Slightly beat together the eggs, milk, salt, and pepper. Pour into the pan.

Bake for 10 minutes or until the eggs begin to set. Sprinkle with cheese and
  chilies. Draw a wide metal spatula across the bottom of the pan several
  times to break up the mixture.

Bake 5 minutes more, or until the desired doneness. Serve with sauce if
  using. Garnish with tomato slices.

PER SERVING (EXCLUDING UNKNOWN ITEMS): 274 calories; 19 g fat (64.4% calories
from fat); 18 g protein; 6 g carbohydrate; trace dietary fiber; 452 mg cholesterol; 663 mg
sodium.

Lunch

SERVES 4

1 large leek, cut in half lengthwise and then crosswise into thin slices

2 whole skinless and boneless chicken breasts, cut into small cubes

1 clove garlic, peeled and crushed

1 large firm, ripe red tomato, peeled, seeded, and chopped

2 small zucchini, washed and cut into small cubes

1 tablespoon fresh tarragon

2 tablespoons chopped Italian parsley

2 ounces reduced-fat Havarti cheese, grated

1 cup finely ground whole wheat bread crumbs

Salt and freshly ground pepper

Extra virgin olive oil

2 large sweet bell peppers, red or yellow, cut in half lengthwise, cored, and seeded

Preheat the oven to 350°F.

In a colander, rinse the leek slices well under warm water to remove grit. In a large bowl, combine the leek, chicken, garlic, tomato, zucchini, tarragon, parsley, cheese, and ½ cup bread crumbs. Add salt and pepper to taste. Toss with ¼ cup olive oil.

Grease the bottom of an ovenproof dish with 1 tablespoon olive oil.

Stuff the pepper halves with the chicken-vegetable mixture, top with the remaining ½ cup bread crumbs, and place in the baking dish. Drizzle olive oil over each stuffed pepper.

Bake in the upper third of the oven until the peppers are tender (45 minutes).

Remove from the oven and moisten with juices from the pan. Serve immediately or at room temperature.

PER SERVING (EXCLUDING UNKNOWN ITEMS): 447 calories; 23 g fat (44.7% calories from fat); 37 g protein; 25 g carbohydrate; 5 g dietary fiber; 90 mg cholesterol; 389 mg sodium.

• STEAMED SEA BASS WITH BABY BOK CHOY AND • SHIITAKE MUSHROOMS IN CITRUS-SOY BROTH

SERVES 4

Miso paste (available in the Japanese section of most grocery stores) gives this dish a wonderful gourmet touch.

3 tablespoons low-sodium soy sauce
One 2-inch piece of ginger root,
    shredded and juice squeezed out
2 teaspoons lime juice
6 heads baby bok choy

2 thick sea bass fillets
2 teaspoons miso or substitute kosher
    salt
8 ounces shiitake mushrooms (fresh, not
    dried), thinly sliced

To make the broth: Combine the soy sauce, ginger root juice, and lime juice in a saucepan and slowly heat until warm.

Place a steamer basket or insert in a large pot filled with simmering water. Pull off the leaves from the baby bok choy, cut off the very bottom part of the stem from each leaf, and rinse well. Place them in the steamer and steam until soft (1–2 minutes) and divide them into two equal portions.

Pat each sea bass fillet dry and coat the tops with a thin layer of miso or salt to taste. Spread half of the baby bok choy leaves on the bottom of the steamer basket and cover with the shiitake mushrooms. Place the fillets on top and cover them with the remaining leaves.

Bring the water to a steady boil and steam the fish until barely translucent in the center, 12–15 minutes depending on the thickness of the fish. Remove from the steamer, arrange on top of the bok choy leaves and mushrooms, and drizzle with the warm citrus-soy broth.

PER SERVING (EXCLUDING UNKNOWN ITEMS): 274 calories; 2 g fat (6.9% calories from fat); 20 g protein; 51 g carbohydrate; 8 g dietary fiber; 26 mg cholesterol; 677 mg sodium.

TURKEY BURGERS WITH BASIL AIOLI AND SPINACH

SERVES 4

Basil mayonnaise is delicious when teamed with a juicy hamburger on a crusty roll.

1 pound ground turkey

3 tablespoons onion, finely chopped

1 clove garlic, peeled and crushed

¾ teaspoon salt

¼ teaspoon pepper

4 whole wheat buns

1 cup packed spinach leaves

4 tomato slices

Basil Aioli Mayonnaise:

3 tablespoons reduced-calorie
  mayonnaise

1 tablespoon chopped fresh
  basil

1 teaspoon Dijon-style mustard

In a medium bowl, combine the ground turkey, onion, garlic, salt, and pepper, mixing lightly but thoroughly. Shape into four ½-inch-thick patties.

Heat a large nonstick skillet or a grill pan over medium heat until hot. Place the patties in the skillet and cook for 7 to 8 minutes, or until fully cooked, turning once.

While the patties are cooking, make the basil mayonnaise by combining the ingredients in a small bowl.

Divide the spinach and tomato slices among the four buns. Place a burger on each tomato and add 1 tablespoon basil mayonnaise. Top with the other half of the roll.

PER SERVING (EXCLUDING UNKNOWN ITEMS): 350 calories; 15 g fat (38.5% calories from fat); 25 g protein; 27 g carbohydrate; 4 g dietary fiber; 93 mg cholesterol; 753 mg sodium.

• SWEET AND SOUR TOM YUM SOUP WITH GINGER • AND STRAW MUSHROOMS

SERVES 4

Although this recipe is vegetarian, you could add cooked skinless and boneless chicken breasts if you like.

2 quarts vegetable stock

2 stalks lemongrass, sliced into
2-inch pieces

4 Kaffir lime leaves (optional)

One 1-inch piece of ginger root, peeled and sliced

2 chili peppers, sliced and seeded if you want the dish milder

2 tablespoons fish sauce

One 8-ounce can straw mushrooms, rinsed and halved

Juice of 2 limes

2 green onions, sliced

1 handful fresh cilantro leaves, chopped

Bring the chicken stock to a boil in a saucepan over medium heat.

Add the lemongrass, Kaffir lime leaves if using, ginger, and chilies.

Lower the heat to medium-low, cover, and simmer for 15 minutes to let the spices infuse the broth.

Uncover and add the fish sauce and mushrooms. Simmer for 5 minutes.

Remove from the heat and add the lime juice, green onions, and cilantro.

Taste for salt and spices. You should have an equal balance of spicy, salty, and sour.

Note: The lemongrass and lime leaves are for flavor only and should be avoided when eating the soup.

PER SERVING (EXCLUDING UNKNOWN ITEMS): 149 calories; 2 g fat (13.2% calories from fat); 5 g protein; 25 g carbohydrate; 1 g dietary fiber; 1 mg cholesterol; 4451 mg sodium.

SERVES 4

This is a refreshing lunch or supper with a sweet, natural crunch.

4 large baking apples to make cups	2 cups chopped celery
⅔ cup golden raisins	¼ cup reduced-fat mayonnaise
1 cup apple juice	1 tablespoon fresh lemon juice
4 large apples, coarsely chopped	½ cup coarsely chopped walnuts

To make apple cups, slice the tops off each baking apple and hollow it out
with a melon baller or knife until about ½ inch thick.

Soak the raisins in apple juice until slightly plumped, then drain.

Toss the chopped apples, celery, raisins, mayonnaise, lemon juice, and
walnuts in a mixing bowl. Fill each apple cup with the salad.

PER SERVING (EXCLUDING UNKNOWN ITEMS): 450 calories; 21 g fat (38.7% calories
from fat); 6 g protein; 69 g carbohydrate; 10 g dietary fiber; 8 mg cholesterol; 60 mg
sodium.

· ASPARAGUS WITH POACHED EGG AND · SAUTÉED MUSHROOMS

SERVES 4

This is a popular lunch or light supper in Europe during the spring asparagus season, and it may be eaten at room temperature. Green asparagus may be used instead of white.

24 spears asparagus, tough
   parts trimmed
4 large eggs
Extra-virgin olive oil
2 tablespoons white wine vinegar
Salt and pepper to taste
2 cups wild or cultivated mushrooms
   (assorted), sliced

6 tablespoons Worcestershire sauce
6 tablespoons low-sodium soy sauce
4 tablespoons yellow onion, minced
2 cups white wine
2 tablespoons fresh oregano

Plunge the asparagus spears into rapidly boiling water for 1 minute, drain, and divide evenly among serving plates.

Poach the eggs in simmering water (see page 163).

Place an egg on each serving of asparagus, drizzle lightly with olive oil, and season with salt and pepper.

Wipe the mushrooms with a damp paper towel. Heat 1 tablespoon of olive oil in a sauté pan over medium heat, add the mushrooms, and sauté until they've given off liquid and begin to dry out, about 5 minutes.

Add the remaining ingredients and simmer gently about 15 minutes.

Serve on the same plate with the egg and asparagus.

PER SERVING (EXCLUDING UNKNOWN ITEMS): 402 calories; 26 g fat (68.7% calories from fat); 11 g protein; 15 g carbohydrate; 3 g dietary fiber; 212 mg cholesterol; 1200 mg sodium.

WISCONSIN "WORKS" TURKEY BURGERS WITH
CHEDDAR AND CARAMELIZED SWEET ONIONS

SERVES 4

Mixing the onions and cheese into the meat patties while cooking adds a delicious twist to an American classic.

2 large onions, peeled and sliced	4 ounces reduced-fat
Extra-virgin olive oil	cheddar cheese, grated
1 pound ground turkey	2 tablespoons Worcestershire sauce
8 ounces mushrooms, chopped	1 tablespoon Dijon mustard
1 medium onion, peeled and	1 egg yolk
chopped	4 whole wheat buns

To make the caramelized onions: Pour enough olive oil to coat the bottom of a heavy skillet plus about 1 tablespoon more. Heat the skillet on high until the oil is very hot but not smoking. Add the sliced onions and turn them with a spatula every 8 to 10 minutes. Continue until all the onion slices have reached a dark, rich brown color, about 40 minutes. After 25 to 30 minutes, add a little bit of water to deglaze the pan and combine the glaze with the onions. Set aside when done.

To make burgers: Combine the ground turkey, mushrooms, chopped onion, cheddar cheese, Worcestershire sauce, mustard, and egg yolk. Mix until well incorporated, and then shape into four small patties.

Heat a cast-iron skillet over high heat and brush the pan lightly with olive oil. Cook each patty for 3–4 minutes per side. Add ¼ cup water, cover the skillet, and cook 3–4 minutes more.

Check the internal temperature of the meat with an instant-read thermometer; it should read at least 135°F.

Serve topped with caramelized onions on brioche buns with desired condiments.

PER SERVING (EXCLUDING UNKNOWN ITEMS): 455 calories; 18 g fat (37.0% calories from fat); 35 g protein; 36 g carbohydrate; 5 g dietary fiber; 149 mg cholesterol; 577 mg sodium.

• SPICY LONE STAR TURKEY CHILI •

SERVES 4

1 tablespoon canola oil

1 medium yellow onion, peeled
   and chopped

2 cloves garlic, peeled and minced

2 teaspoons chili powder

1 teaspoon dried oregano

1 teaspoon cumin

½ teaspoon red pepper flakes

½ teaspoon hot pepper sauce (or more
   to taste)

1 can diced green chilies

1 pound canned tomatoes, chopped

1⅓ teaspoons salt

2⅔ cups chopped cooked turkey

Heat the oil in a skillet, add the onions and garlic, and cook until limp. Add
   the chili powder, oregano, cumin, red pepper flakes, hot pepper sauce,
   green chilies, tomatoes, and salt. Simmer for 15 minutes. Add the cooked
   turkey and simmer for 10 minutes more.

PER SERVING (EXCLUDING UNKNOWN ITEMS): 232 calories; 9 g fat (33.4% calories from
fat); 29 g protein; 9 g carbohydrate; 2 g dietary fiber; 71 mg cholesterol; 898 mg sodium.

· ASIAN BEEF SALAD WITH SOY VINAIGRETTE ·

SERVES 4

This recipe works well for any module except INDUCTION.

For the beef:

12 ounces sirloin or filet mignon
   steak, cut into thin strips
1½ tablespoons soy sauce
1½ tablespoons canola oil
2 cloves garlic, minced
Black pepper

For the salad:
¼ cup canola oil
1 teaspoon wasabi powder

1 tablespoon low-sodium soy sauce
1½ tablespoons rice vinegar
1 teaspoon sesame oil
2 cups assorted lettuce leaves such as
   spring mix
2 large carrots, peeled and grated
1 bunch green scallions, sliced
1 tablespoon toasted sesame seeds for
   garnish

In a bowl, combine the steak, soy sauce, canola oil, garlic, and pepper. Let
marinate for 15 minutes. Heat a nonstick skillet over moderately high heat
until it is hot. Add the steak, marinade, and salt, and cook, stirring, just
until the meat is no longer pink. Be careful not to overcook. With a slotted
spoon transfer the steak to a plate.

To make the salad, whisk together in a small bowl the canola oil, wasabi
powder, soy sauce, vinegar, and sesame oil. Save a little for garnish and
toss the remaining vinaigrette with the beef, lettuce, carrots, and scallions.
Garnish with the sesame seeds.

PER SERVING (EXCLUDING UNKNOWN ITEMS): 240 calories; 20 g fat (72.6% calories
from fat); 3 g protein; 14 g carbohydrate; 4 g dietary fiber; 0 mg cholesterol; 580 mg
sodium.

· BABY MÂCHE SALAD WITH BLOOD ORANGE · SEGMENTS, ROASTED GOLDEN BEETS, GOAT CHEESE, AND "WHOLE CITRUS VINAIGRETTE"

SERVES 4

This is a delicious salad that combines sweet and bitter flavors with creamy and firm textures. If any ingredients are unavailable, you may substitute similar ones.

2 blood oranges
1 shallot, peeled and thinly sliced
Salt to taste
2 tablespoons extra-virgin olive oil

5 cups mâche or romaine lettuce
2 roasted golden beets, thinly sliced
4 ounces goat cheese, crumbled

To make the "Whole Citrus Vinaigrette": In a food processor or juicer, puree the whole blood oranges, complete with rind, and strain. Add the shallots and salt to the juice, in a small bowl. Whisk in the olive oil.

Toss the lettuce, beets, and goat cheese in a large salad bowl and drizzle with the vinaigrette.

PER SERVING (EXCLUDING UNKNOWN ITEMS): 228 calories; 17 g fat (65.6% calories from fat); 10 g protein; 10 g carbohydrate; 2 g dietary fiber; 30 mg cholesterol; 104 mg sodium.

· BANANA LEAF-WRAPPED SEASONAL FRESH FISH · WITH CHIPOTLE-CITRUS BUTTER AND SWEET POTATO PUREE

SERVES 4

The banana leaf imparts a delicious flavor while steaming. If it is unavailable, use parchment paper instead.

2 tablespoons unsalted butter, softened

1 tablespoon adobo sauce (available in the Mexican section of the grocery store)

Juice and zest of 1 orange

Juice and zest of 1 lime

4 medium sweet potatoes

6 tablespoons low-sodium chicken broth

Salt and pepper (optional)

1 package banana leaves

2 pounds seasonal fresh fish fillet, cut into 4 pieces

½ cup white wine

To make the chipotle-citrus butter: Mix the softened butter with the adobo sauce and citrus juices and zests. Shape the butter mixture into a log and chill until firm.

To make the sweet potato puree: Peel the sweet potatoes and cut into 1-inch pieces. In a small saucepan, boil the potatoes in salted water for 15 minutes, or until very tender, and drain well in a colander. In a food processor, puree the potatoes with the chicken broth until smooth. Add salt and pepper if desired.

To make the fish: Preheat the oven to 375°F. Cut each banana leaf into 2-inch-wide strips. Place each piece of fish in the center of a banana leaf. Add a pinch of salt and a teaspoon of the chipotle-citrus butter to each piece. Roll up each piece tightly in the banana leaf and place, folded side down, on a cookie sheet lined with parchment paper. Bake for approximately 10 minutes or until the fish is cooked through. To serve, open each banana leaf to expose the fish and dab with the citrus butter. Add a side of sweet potato puree.

PER SERVING (EXCLUDING UNKNOWN ITEMS): 447 calories; 10 g fat (20.6% calories from fat); 44 g protein; 39 g carbohydrate; 5 g dietary fiber; 113 mg cholesterol; 237 mg sodium.

· WALNUT SALAD WITH APPLE CIDER VINAIGRETTE ·

SERVES 4

This is a very quick salad to assemble when you're short on time.

2 heads frisée lettuce, cored and
    leaves separated, or 2 cups
    mesclun mix
3 Granny Smith apples, thinly sliced
½ cup walnuts
¾ cup golden raisins

¼ cup cider vinegar
½ cup canola oil
1 tablespoon Dijon mustard
2 tablespoons honey
Salt and pepper to taste

Mix the frisée or mesclun with the apple, walnuts, and golden raisins in a
    large bowl.
For the vinaigrette, combine the cider vinegar, canola oil, mustard, and
    honey, and season with salt and pepper. Whisk together until emulsified.

PER SERVING (EXCLUDING UNKNOWN ITEMS): 464 calories; 29 g fat (52.8% calories
from fat); 2 g protein; 56 g carbohydrate; 5 g dietary fiber; 2 mg cholesterol; 77 mg
sodium.

· CARROT AND SAFFRON SOUP ·

This soup makes a wonderful lunch.

1 pound carrots	Water
2 stalks celery	1 cup white wine
1 pound leeks	2 teaspoons salt
1 tablespoon canola oil	½ teaspoon white pepper
½ teaspoon saffron threads	3 cups skim milk

Peel and grate the carrots. Finely chop the celery. Slit the leeks and wash well under cold water, separating the leaves and making sure all sand is removed. Shake off the water and then slice the leeks finely.

Place the canola oil in a heavy saucepan and add the leeks. Stir to coat with the oil and then turn the heat very low. Cover the pan and sweat the leeks for about 8 minutes, until soft but not brown. Add the carrots and celery, stir well, cover, and cook 5 minutes more.

Meanwhile, toast the saffron in a small, dry pan for about 1 minute, to make it brittle enough to grind to a powder in a mortar and pestle. Dissolve the ground saffron in 2 tablespoons hot water and add to the vegetables in the pan. Add 3 cups water, wine, salt, and pepper.

Cook, covered, for 10 minutes, or until the carrots are very tender. Add the milk and heat through without boiling. Taste and correct the seasoning.

Serve hot.

PER SERVING (EXCLUDING UNKNOWN ITEMS): 213 calories; 4 g fat (20.4% calories from fat); 8 g protein; 28 g carbohydrate; 4 g dietary fiber; 3 mg cholesterol; 1106 mg sodium.

• CHICKEN LETTUCE WRAPS WITH SPICY • CHILI-GARLIC DIPPING SAUCE

SERVES 4

1 pound skinless chicken breast

Salt and pepper to taste

2 tablespoons canola oil

2 tablespoons minced ginger root

4 cloves garlic, peeled and minced

1 large red bell pepper, seeded and very thinly sliced

½ cup shredded cabbage

½ cup shredded carrot

3 scallions, sliced

½ cup plum sauce

2 cups basil leaves

1 tablespoon fish sauce

½ head iceberg lettuce, each leaf cut in half

½ cucumber, peeled and chopped

Dipping Sauce:

1½ tablespoons low-sodium soy sauce

1 tablespoon seasoned rice vinegar

1 tablespoon chili sauce (Asian style)

1 teaspoon hot chili oil

2 cloves garlic, minced

To make the chicken: Thinly slice it into strips and sprinkle with salt and pepper. Heat a large skillet until it is very hot but not smoking. Add the canola oil and then the chicken. Cook for 2 minutes, stirring constantly, and then add the ginger, garlic, pepper, cabbage, carrots, and scallions. Stir-fry 2 minutes more. Add the plum sauce and toss for 1 minute. Add the basil and cook until the leaves wilt. Add the fish sauce and toss.

Transfer the cooked chicken and vegetables to a bowl.

To make the dipping sauce: Combine the soy sauce, vinegar, chili-garlic sauce, and hot chili oil in a medium bowl. Mix well and set aside.

To serve: Place spoonfuls of chicken and some cucumber on a piece of lettuce. Fold the lettuce over and eat like a small taco.

PER SERVING (EXCLUDING UNKNOWN ITEMS): 274 calories; 10 g fat (33.3% calories from fat); 24 g protein; 22 g carbohydrate; 3 g dietary fiber; 53 mg cholesterol; 437 mg sodium.

• ORGANIC MIXED GREENS WITH ROASTED PEACHES, • GOAT CHEESE CROUTONS, AND SHERRY VINAIGRETTE

SERVES 4

2 tablespoons sherry vinegar

¼ cup extra-virgin olive oil

1 shallot, peeled and minced

1 tablespoon honey

3 semi-firm fresh peaches

4 slices whole wheat bread, crusts
removed

6 ounces goat cheese

Salt and pepper to taste

2 bags organic mixed greens

For the vinaigrette, combine the sherry vinegar, olive oil, shallot, and honey until well mixed. Set aside.

Roast the peaches whole in a 300°F oven for 30 minutes. Let the peaches cool slightly, then slice and set aside.

Toast the bread slices on a baking sheet in a 350°F oven for 8–10 minutes or until golden brown and crisp. Brush each slice with olive oil and then crumble the goat cheese over each slice.

Dress the greens with the vinaigrette, salt, and pepper. Arrange the peaches around the salad and top with the croutons.

PER SERVING (EXCLUDING UNKNOWN ITEMS): 436 calories; 30 g fat (60.1% calories from fat); 17 g protein; 28 g carbohydrate; 4 g dietary fiber; 45 mg cholesterol; 298 mg sodium.

· GRILLED GLOBE ZUCCHINI "STEAK" WITH QUINOA ·

SERVES 4

Quinoa is an extremely healthy whole-germ South American grain. If unavailable, substitute any other whole grain or unpolished brown rice.

1 cup quinoa
2½ cups vegetable broth
8 large globe zucchini (big round shape) or 8 medium-sized regular zucchini

1 tablespoon extra-virgin olive oil
Salt and pepper to taste
1 tablespoon balsamic vinegar

Cook the quinoa in the vegetable broth until it fluffs up, about 15 minutes. Stir occasionally.

Trim off the ends of each zucchini to create 8 thick "steak"-size portions. Drizzle the zucchini "steaks" with olive oil and season with salt and pepper. (If using regular zucchini, cut in half lengthwise to make 2 "steaks.")

Heat a grill pan until lightly smoking. Cook each "steak" for 5 minutes on each side. (If using regular zucchini, cook each "steak" for 2 minutes on each side.) Drizzle with balsamic vinegar.

PER SERVING (EXCLUDING UNKNOWN ITEMS): 346 calories; 9 g fat (21.7% calories from fat); 14 g protein; 57 g carbohydrate; 9 g dietary fiber; 2 mg cholesterol; 1037 mg sodium.

• HERB-ROASTED CHICKEN BREAST WITH PAN • JUICES AND ROOT VEGETABLES

SERVES 4

4 skinless split chicken breasts

3 cloves fresh garlic, peeled

1 teaspoon fresh thyme

2 tablespoons fresh rosemary

1 teaspoon salt

Freshly ground black pepper

1 tablespoon extra-virgin olive oil

1½ tablespoons red wine vinegar

2 parsnips

3 carrots

2 turnips

Olive oil

Garlic powder

To make the chicken: Finely mince the garlic, thyme, and rosemary leaves. Mix in salt, ½ teaspoon pepper, olive oil, and vinegar. Rub the mixture on all sides of the chicken.

Preheat the oven to 350°F.

Place the chicken on a rack in a roasting pan. Lightly brush the chicken with olive oil. Bake uncovered for 30 minutes or until the juices run clear when the chicken is pierced with a fork.

To make the root vegetables: Peel and cut the parsnips, carrots, and turnips into large chunks. Arrange in a roasting pan and season with olive oil, salt, pepper, and garlic powder. Roast until tender. Check the vegetables for doneness after 25 minutes and then every 10 minutes thereafter.

PER SERVING (EXCLUDING UNKNOWN ITEMS): 303 calories; 5 g fat (16.1% calories from fat); 30 g protein; 34 g carbohydrate; 9 g dietary fiber; 68 mg cholesterol; 626 mg sodium.

• ORGANIC MIXED GREENS SALAD WITH ROASTED •
BUTTERNUT SQUASH, RED AND GOLD BEETS,
GOAT CHEESE, AND AGED BALSAMIC DRIZZLE

SERVES 4

This salad is lightly dressed with aged balsamic but no oil. It is not needed thanks to the creamy beets and squash, which are loaded with fiber.

4 red beets

4 gold beets

Water

Salt and pepper

1 butternut squash, peeled and
  cut into 1-inch dice

1 pound mixed greens

4 ounces goat cheese, crumbled

Aged balsamic vinegar

Preheat the oven to 400°F.

To roast the beets: Scrub and trim the beets. Line a baking pan with foil and add the beets, water, salt, and pepper. Cover and roast in the oven for 45 minutes, then remove and let cool. Peel the beets and cut into wedges.

To roast the squash: Toss the squash with salt and pepper. Roast uncovered for 25 minutes on a baking sheet that has been coated in nonstick cooking spray. Remove and allow to cool.

To assemble the salad: Toss all the ingredients including the mixed greens and goat cheese. Drizzle with balsamic vinegar and serve.

PER SERVING (EXCLUDING UNKNOWN ITEMS): 420 calories; 11 g fat (21.5% calories from fat); 19 g protein; 72 g carbohydrate; 16 g dietary fiber; 30 mg cholesterol; 271 mg sodium.

· CHINESE CHICKEN SALAD WITH NAPA CABBAGE, · SNAP PEAS, AND SWEET AND SOUR RICE WINE DRESSING

SERVES 4

2½ tablespoons low-sodium
   soy sauce
1½ teaspoons sesame oil
1 pound skinless boneless chicken
   breast
⅓ head napa cabbage, thinly
   shredded
⅛ head red cabbage, shredded
1 large carrot, shredded
1 cup sugar snap peas
2 scallions, trimmed and thinly sliced,
   green portion included

One 8-ounce can water chestnuts,
   sliced
1 orange or clementine, sectioned
¼ cup rice wine vinegar
1 teaspoon minced garlic
1 teaspoon minced ginger
1½ tablespoons canola oil
1½ tablespoons brown sugar
1 teaspoon chili sauce
¼ cup sliced almonds, toasted

Preheat oven to 350°F.

Combine 1 tablespoon of the soy sauce and ½ teaspoon of the sesame oil. Brush this mixture on the chicken breasts. Arrange in a baking dish and bake until the juices run clear, 13 to 15 minutes. Remove from the oven, cool completely, and cut into ¼-inch slices.

In a large bowl, combine the Napa cabbage, red cabbage, carrot, sugar snap peas, scallions, water chestnuts, orange, and sliced chicken. In a separate bowl, whisk together the remaining 1½ tablespoons of soy sauce, vinegar, garlic, ginger, canola oil, 1 teaspoon sesame oil, the brown sugar, and chili sauce. Pour the dressing over the salad and toss to combine. Divide among the bowls and top each serving with some of the toasted almonds.

PER SERVING (EXCLUDING UNKNOWN ITEMS): 354 calories; 14 g fat (35.5% calories from fat); 30 g protein; 28 g carbohydrate; 5 g dietary fiber; 69 mg cholesterol; 456 mg sodium.

· KICKIN' CABBAGE SOUP ·

SERVES 4

1 tablespoon oil	3 medium carrots, sliced
2 medium onions, diced	1 ham hock
1 medium green cabbage, cored	3 tablespoon wine vinegar
and shredded	½ teaspoon sage
1¼ quart chicken broth	½ teaspoon thyme
3 small potatoes, cubed	Salt and pepper to taste

In a large pot, heat the oil and cook the onions, stirring occasionally, until
softened (about 10 minutes). Add the cabbage and cook, stirring
occasionally, about 15 minutes. Add the chicken broth, potatoes, carrots,
ham hock, vinegar, sage, and thyme. Cover and simmer the soup for 50
minutes. Remove from heat and add salt and pepper as desired.

Chill for 8 hours, then skim the fat from the top of the soup. Reheat and serve.

Dinner

· BLACKENED CHICKEN BREAST ·
WITH BLACK-EYED PEAS AND BRAISED GREENS

SERVES 4

This dish is loaded with protein and fiber, and using frozen peas and greens speeds the cooking.

12 ounces frozen black-eyed peas

2 cups water

1 large chicken or vegetable-flavor bouillon cube

1 small yellow onion, peeled and chopped

1 package frozen collard greens

1 teaspoon minced garlic

12 ounces low-sodium chicken broth

Worcestershire sauce to taste

Tabasco sauce to taste

1 teaspoon paprika

½ teaspoon cayenne pepper

½ teaspoon dried thyme

¼ teaspoon onion powder

½ teaspoon ground cumin

¼ teaspoon salt

¼ teaspoon ground white pepper

2 tablespoons canola oil

4 skinless boneless chicken breasts

Combine the peas, water, bouillon cube, and yellow onion in a large saucepan and bring to a boil. Reduce the heat and simmer for 30 minutes or until tender.

While the peas are cooking, combine the collard greens, garlic, broth, Worcestershire sauce, and Tabasco sauce in a saucepan and cook over medium heat until tender.

Rinse the chicken breasts and pat dry. Preheat the oven to 350°F. Combine the herbs, salt, and pepper, and rub the mixture on one side of each chicken breast.

In a cast-iron skillet or heavy nonstick pan, heat the canola oil over high heat. It may take up to 10 minutes to reach desired heat. Make sure the oil is not too hot or smoking.

Place the chicken in the hot pan, seasoned side down, and cook for 1
   minute. Turn and cook 1 minute on the other side. Place the breasts
   on a lightly greased cookie sheet and put in the preheated oven for 5 to
   10 minutes, or until the meat is no longer pink and the juices run clear.
For each serving, place a small mound of greens on each plate and top with
   the peas and a chicken breast.

PER SERVING (EXCLUDING UNKNOWN ITEMS): 548 calories; 11 g fat (18.5% calories
from fat); 73 g protein; 41 g carbohydrate; 13 g dietary fiber; 137 mg cholesterol; 570 mg
sodium.

• BEEF SATAY SKEWERS WITH PEANUT • DIPPING SAUCE

SERVES 4

This recipe is high in protein and unsaturated fats and perfect if you are entertaining while dieting.

1 pound flank steak, cut against the grain into thin, wide strips
½ cup teriyaki marinade
1 tablespoon peeled and minced ginger
1 tablespoon peeled and minced garlic
Salt
2 teaspoons peanut oil
1 cup dry-roasted unsalted peanuts

2 large shallots, peeled and sliced
2 cloves garlic, peeled and sliced
3 chili peppers, seeded and minced
3 Kaffir lime leaves sliced into thin strips (optional)
½ cup light coconut milk
1 cup water
2 tablespoons low-sodium soy sauce
Pepper to taste
Juice of 1 lemon

To make the beef satay: Place the beef strips in a medium-size bowl and pour the teriyaki marinade over them. Add the ginger, garlic, and 1 teaspoon salt, then stir to combine. Place the strips on skewers and grill for 2 minutes per side.

To make the peanut sauce: In a skillet coated with half of the peanut oil, sauté the peanuts until golden brown, about 4 to 6 minutes, drain on paper towels to cool. Transfer to a food processor and grind finely. Coat the skillet with the remaining peanut oil. Add the shallots, garlic, and peppers, and stir for 2 minutes, until fragrant. Add the Kaffir lime leaves if using, coconut milk, water, soy sauce, and peanuts, and season with salt and pepper. Simmer for 15 to 20 minutes, until the desired consistency is reached; it should be similar to pesto. Add the lemon juice and check for seasoning.

Serve the beef skewers with the peanut sauce.

PER SERVING (EXCLUDING UNKNOWN ITEMS): 525 calories; 34 g fat (55.9% calories from fat); 33 g protein; 27 g carbohydrate; 4 g dietary fiber; 58 mg cholesterol; 2045 mg sodium.

• QUICK WHITE BEAN AND TURKEY CHILI • WITH SWISS CHARD

SERVES 4

This dish is packed with protein and flavor and tastes as hearty as it looks.

1 tablespoon extra-virgin olive oil
1 medium yellow onion, finely
   chopped
3 cloves garlic, minced
1 bunch Swiss chard leaves,
   coarsely chopped
1 can great northern beans
1 can white kidney (cannellini) beans

2 cups low-sodium chicken broth
1 teaspoon ground cumin
½ teaspoon dried oregano
12 ounces cooked turkey breast,
   chopped
Salt and pepper to taste
4 tablespoons fat-free sour cream

In a large stockpot, heat the olive oil over medium heat and add the onion
   and garlic. Cook for a few minutes, until tender. Add the Swiss chard and
   cook until wilted, about 5 minutes.
Stir in the beans, broth, cumin, and oregano. Bring to a boil, reduce the heat,
   cover the pot, and simmer for 10 minutes. Add the turkey, cover, and
   simmer 10 minutes more. Adjust the seasonings if desired.
Ladle into soup bowls and garnish with sour cream.

PER SERVING (EXCLUDING UNKNOWN ITEMS): 557 calories; 12 g fat (18.6% calories
from fat); 54 g protein; 65 g carbohydrate; 18 g dietary fiber; 65 mg cholesterol;
122 mg sodium.

• BEEF AND VEGETABLE STIR-FRY WITH BROWN RICE •

SERVES 4

2 tablespoons low-sodium soy
  sauce
2 tablespoons rice vinegar
1 tablespoon sesame oil
⅓ teaspoon five-spice powder
1 pound flank steak, cut into
  ¼-inch strips
¼ cup water
⅔ teaspoon cornstarch
1 teaspoon peanut oil
1 tablespoon sesame seeds, toasted

2 teaspoons ginger root, peeled and
  minced
2 cloves garlic, peeled and minced
1½ cups sliced red bell peppers
1 cup fresh or frozen blanched shelled
  edamame
⅔ cup sliced Shiitake mushroom caps
10 ounces corn (canned, use fresh if
  available), drained
⅓ cup sliced green onions
2 cups cooked brown rice

Combine half the soy sauce, half the vinegar, the sesame oil, and the five-spice powder in a medium bowl, stirring with a whisk. Add the beef and toss to coat. Let stand for 10 minutes. Remove the beef from the bowl and discard the marinade.

Combine the remaining soy sauce and vinegar, water, and cornstarch, stirring with a whisk.

Heat the peanut oil in a large nonstick skillet over medium-high heat. Add the sesame seeds, ginger, and garlic, and stir-fry for 30 seconds. Add the bell pepper, edamame, mushrooms, and corn, and stir-fry for 2 minutes. Add the beef and the cornstarch mixture and stir-fry for 3 minutes, or until the sauce thickens.

Remove from the heat and stir in the onions.

Serve over steamed brown rice.

PER SERVING (EXCLUDING UNKNOWN ITEMS): 608 calories; 23 g fat (32.3% calories from fat); 39 g protein; 68 g carbohydrate; 10 g dietary fiber; 58 mg cholesterol; 498 mg sodium.

• WHOLE WHEAT NEAPOLITAN-STYLE PIZZA WITH • HOMEMADE TOMATO SAUCE, TURKEY SAUSAGE, AND FRESH MOZZARELLA

SERVES 4

This traditional-style pizza is loaded with fiber, calcium, lycopene, and other nutrients.

Pizza Dough:
¾ cup water (105°F to 115°F)
1 envelope active dry yeast
Olive oil
2 cups whole wheat flour
1 teaspoon brown sugar
¾ teaspoon kosher salt

Tomato Sauce:
1 medium yellow onion, diced
2 tablespoons extra-virgin olive oil
4 cloves garlic, peeled and thinly
    sliced
½ cup fresh basil

½ cup red wine
1½ pounds fresh tomato, diced
Salt and pepper to taste
4½ tablespoons fresh parsley

Pizza:
Flour or cornmeal for coating the pan
12 ounces ripe tomato, sliced
6 ounces turkey breakfast sausage,
    crumbled and cooked
3 cloves garlic, minced
2 fresh basil leaves, sliced thinly
12 ounces buffalo mozzarella,
    diced

To make the pizza dough: Pour the warm water into a small bowl and stir in
    the yeast. Let stand until the yeast dissolves, about 5 minutes.
Brush a large bowl lightly with olive oil.
Mix the flour, sugar, and salt in a food processor. Add the yeast mixture and
    3 tablespoons olive oil; process until the dough forms a sticky ball.
Transfer to a lightly floured surface and knead the dough about 1 minute,
    until smooth. Add more flour by tablespoonfuls if the dough is very sticky.
Transfer to the prepared bowl and then turn the dough in the bowl to coat
    with oil. Cover the bowl with plastic wrap and let the dough rise in a warm
    draft-free area until doubled in volume, about 1 hour.
To make the tomato sauce: Sauté the onion in olive oil in a covered pan over
    low heat for 10–12 minutes.

Add the garlic and basil, cover again, and cook for another 5 minutes. Uncover, add the wine, and cook until reduced by about half.

Add the tomatoes, salt, and pepper and simmer for a minimum of 15 minutes. Cooking longer reduces the sauce further and intensifies the flavor.

Add the fresh parsley at the end.

To make the pizza: Preheat the oven to 350°F. Press the dough into a disk about 8 inches in diameter. Slide the pastry disk onto an edgeless pizza pan coated with flour or cornmeal. Make sure the pastry disk is thin.

Spread the tomato sauce on the pastry disk and add the tomato slices, cooked turkey sausage, and minced garlic.

Spread the diced buffalo mozzarella over the tomatoes.

Bake the pizza for 20–25 minutes, or until the crust is browned and the cheese has melted.

Scatter the basil leaves over the pizza as you take it out of the oven.

PER SERVING (EXCLUDING UNKNOWN ITEMS): 574 calories; 29 g fat (45.4% calories from fat); 18 g protein; 62 g carbohydrate; 11 g dietary fiber; 34 mg cholesterol; 687 mg sodium.

· PESTO-CRUSTED CHICKEN BREAST WITH · EGGPLANT CAPONATA

SERVES 4

Caponata is a delicious relish that can be prepared in advance and served at room temperature. Prepared caponata may be used in place of homemade.

4 ounces prepared pesto sauce

2 tablespoons chopped walnuts

2 tablespoons lemon juice

1 teaspoon grated lemon peel

4 boneless skinless chicken breasts

2 teaspoons extra-virgin olive oil

2 medium eggplants, chopped

1 tablespoon extra-virgin olive oil

Salt and pepper to taste

½ medium yellow onion, peeled and chopped

3 cloves garlic, peeled and minced

2 large Roma tomatoes, chopped

2 tablespoons pine nuts, toasted

2 tablespoons red wine vinegar

Preheat the oven to 425°F. Combine the pesto, chopped walnuts, lemon juice, and grated lemon peel in a food processor and pulse until just combined. Place the chicken breasts on a large baking pan. Coat the chicken with the pesto mixture and drizzle with olive oil. Bake until the chicken is cooked through, about 30 minutes.

Bake the eggplants while the chicken is baking. Toss the chopped eggplant with half of the olive oil and season with salt and pepper. Spread the eggplant in a single layer on another baking pan and bake in the oven for 20 minutes or until tender.

Meanwhile, sauté the onion and garlic in the remaining olive oil over medium heat stirring occasionally, until the onions are translucent. Add the tomatoes and eggplants and continue to cook for 3 to 4 minutes. Add the pine nuts and vinegar, and cook for 8 to 10 minutes, stirring often, until the caponata is nicely blended and cooked.

When serving, top each chicken breast with a generous serving of caponata.

PER SERVING (EXCLUDING UNKNOWN ITEMS): 593 calories; 28 g fat (41.5% calories from fat); 65 g protein; 23 g carbohydrate; 8 g dietary fiber; 146 mg cholesterol; 373 mg sodium.

PROVENÇALE VEGETABLE SOUP WITH SAFFRON, LEEKS, BABY GREEN BEANS, AND BASIL PESTO

SERVES 4

1½ tablespoons extra-virgin olive oil

1 medium yellow onion, peeled and chopped

1½ cups chopped leeks

1 medium russet potato, peeled and cubed

2 cups finely chopped carrots

1 tablespoon salt

⅔ teaspoon ground black pepper

2 quarts vegetable stock

1 teaspoon saffron threads

5 basil stems, leaves removed

8 ounces haricots verts (baby green beans), ends removed and cut in half

½ cup pesto sauce

Heat the olive oil in a large stockpot. Add the onions and sauté over low heat for 10 minutes, or until the onions are translucent. Add the leeks, potatoes, carrots, salt, and pepper, and sauté over medium heat 5 minutes more.

Add the stock, saffron, and basil, bring to a boil, and then simmer uncovered for 30 minutes, or until all the vegetables are tender.

Add the haricots verts, bring to a simmer, and cook 15 minutes more.

To serve: Whisk one-fourth of the pesto into the hot soup and then season to taste. Depending on the saltiness of your chicken stock, you may need to add more salt, up to another tablespoon. Drizzle each bowl with the remaining pesto.

PER SERVING (EXCLUDING UNKNOWN ITEMS): 597 calories; 27 g fat (40.0% calories from fat); 19 g protein; 72 g carbohydrate; 12 g dietary fiber; 14 mg cholesterol; 4902 mg sodium.

· RED LENTIL SOUP WITH BARLEY AND KALE ·

SERVES 4

1 tablespoon extra-virgin olive oil
1 medium yellow onion, peeled
  and chopped
1 carrot, peeled and chopped
2 cloves garlic, peeled and minced
2 teaspoons ground cumin
2 quarts vegetable stock

½ cup pearl barley
½ cup dried red lentils
12 ounces canned tomatoes, diced,
  liquid reserved
2 cups chopped kale
Salt and pepper to taste

Heat the olive oil in a heavy stockpot over medium-high heat. Add the onions and carrots, and sauté until the onions are golden brown, about 10 minutes. Add the garlic and stir for 1 minute. Mix in the cumin and stir for 30 seconds. Add the vegetable stock and barley, and bring to a boil. Lower the heat, cover lightly, and simmer for 25 minutes. Stir in the lentils and tomatoes with their juice. Cover and simmer until the barley and lentils are tender, about 30 minutes. Add kale, cover, and simmer until the kale is tender, about 5 minutes. Stir in dill. Season soup with salt and pepper. Thin with more stock if desired.

PER SERVING (EXCLUDING UNKNOWN ITEMS): 581 calories; 12 g fat (18.4% calories from fat); 24 g protein; 98 g carbohydrate; 20 g dietary fiber; 5 mg cholesterol; 3406 mg sodium.

SALADE NIÇOISE WITH FRESH TUNA, OLIVES, EGG, LETTUCE, AND BABY GREEN BEANS WITH DIJON VINAIGRETTE

SERVES 4

1 pound yellowfin tuna steaks

Salt to taste

Ground black pepper to taste

1 tablespoon extra-virgin olive oil

1½ sprigs rosemary

1 head lettuce, rinsed and patted dry

1 teaspoon minced fresh parsley

1 teaspoon minced fresh tarragon

4 new potatoes, boiled until tender, then sliced

⅓ pound haricots verts (baby green beans), ends trimmed

⅓ pound Roma tomatoes, cut into 1-inch cubes

¼ cup black olives, halved and seeded

¼ cup green olives, halved and seeded

⅓ cup red onion, peeled and thinly sliced

2 hard-boiled eggs, peeled and sliced

Minced fresh herbs for garnish (parsley, tarragon, chives, etc.) (optional)

Dijon Vinaigrette:

½ cup extra-virgin olive oil

1 tablespoon dijon mustard

1 clove garlic, peeled and minced

Salt and pepper to taste

¼ cup red wine vinegar

Arrange the tuna on a cutting board and cut into 4 equal portions. Season each tuna steak with ¼ teaspoon salt and ¼ teaspoon pepper. Heat the olive oil in a large skillet or 2 medium skillets, over medium-high heat. When the oil is hot but not smoking, add the rosemary sprigs and tuna steaks and sear about 30 seconds per side for medium-rare. Remove from the pan and cut the tuna into 1-inch dice.

Tear the lettuce into bite-size pieces and combine with the parsley and tarragon. Add additional salt and pepper as needed. Toss the potatoes and green beans in ¼ cup of dijon vinaigrette. Arrange the lettuce along the side of 4 large plates or 1 serving platter. Spoon the vegetables along the other side. Arrange the diced tuna over the lettuce. Arrange the tomatoes,

(continued)

olives, onions, and eggs on the other sides. Garnish with additional herbs if desired and serve immediately.

For the vinaigrette: Whisk together olive oil, mustard, and garlic with salt and pepper until combined. Slowly whisk in the vinegar until the vinaigrette is emulsified.

PER SERVING (EXCLUDING UNKNOWN ITEMS): 426 calories; 28 g fat (59.8% calories from fat); 33 g protein; 9 g carbohydrate; 3 g dietary fiber; 203 mg cholesterol; 797 mg sodium.

· CHILLED WILD RICE AND TROPICAL FRUIT SALAD ·
WITH CITRUS-GINGER-VANILLA SYRUP

SERVES 4

This recipe also works well with leftover cooked brown rice.

½ cup firmly packed brown sugar

¼ cup lime juice

1 quart water

1 tablespoon unsalted butter

2 pieces crystallized ginger

1 teaspoon vanilla extract

3 tablespoons crystallized ginger, minced

2 cups wild rice

3 cups peeled and diced fresh tropical
    fruit (pineapple, papaya, mango, etc.)

Shredded coconut for garnish

Combine the brown sugar, 1 quart water, lime juice, butter, ginger pieces, and vanilla extract in a heavy medium-size saucepan. Stir over medium heat until the sugar dissolves. Boil gently, stirring frequently, until reduced to 1 cup, about 15 minutes. Cool to lukewarm. Discard the ginger pieces and add the minced ginger. (This can be prepared 1 day ahead. Cover, store at room temperature, and then reheat to lukewarm, whisking occasionally, before serving.)

In a medium-size pot, bring the wild rice and water to a boil. Reduce the heat to low, cover, and simmer until tender, about 35 minutes. Refrigerate until cool.

To serve: Top the rice with tropical fruit, spoon lukewarm sauce over the fruit and rice, and top with coconut.

PER SERVING (EXCLUDING UNKNOWN ITEMS): 489 calories; 4 g fat (7.0% calories from fat); 12 g protein; 106 g carbohydrate; 5 g dietary fiber; 8 mg cholesterol; 44 mg sodium.

• CEDAR PLANK ROASTED WILD SALMON WITH RED • WINE REDUCTION AND WILD MUSHROOM SAUTÉ

SERVES 4

If you do not find a cedar plank at a local kitchen or hardware store, then simply roast the salmon on the foil-lined baking sheet.

Salmon:
1½ pounds salmon fillet
1 tablespoon canola oil
1 tablespoon brown sugar
Salt and pepper to taste

Red Wine Reduction:
4 tablespoons extra-virgin olive oil
2 shallots, peeled and minced
8 cloves garlic, peeled and
   minced
½ cup red wine
½ cup beef or vegetable stock
1 tablespoon unsalted butter

4 tablespoons fresh herbs such as
   Italian parsley, chives, or other
   seasonal herbs

Mushroom Sauté:
2 tablespoons canola oil
6 ounces assorted wild mushrooms
   such as morels, chanterelles,
   porcini, or others in season,
   cleaned and sliced
6 ounces domestic mushrooms,
   cleaned and sliced
Salt and pepper to taste
1 cedar plank, 6 by 14 inches

Preheat the oven to 400°F.

Place the salmon fillet in a long shallow dish. Mix all the other ingredients together and pour over the salmon. Marinate for 30 minutes.

Meanwhile, make the reduction. Heat the olive oil in a saucepan over medium heat. Add the shallots and garlic and sauté for 3 minutes or until translucent. Add the red wine, raise the heat to medium-high, and allow to cook for 1 to 2 minutes. Add the stock and continue to cook until reduced to one-third of its original volume, 15 to 20 minutes. Turn off the heat. Add the butter, and whisk to incorporate it fully. Add fresh herbs and adjust seasonings to taste.

While the sauce is reducing, heat the canola oil in a saucepan over medium-high heat. Add the mushrooms and sauté for 3 minutes per side. Do not disturb the mushrooms while they are cooking so they caramelize.

Place the cedar plank directly on an oven rack and bake for 8–10 minutes. This will lightly toast the wood. Remove the plank from the oven and rub with a thin coating of olive oil while the plank is still hot. Put the salmon directly on a foil-lined baking sheet and place the sheet on the hot plank. Roast on the plank for 10 minutes.

Serve the salmon topped with mushrooms and accompany with the reduction.

PER SERVING (EXCLUDING UNKNOWN ITEMS): 516 calories; 33 g fat (60.2% calories from fat); 37 g protein; 13 g carbohydrate; 1 g dietary fiber; 97 mg cholesterol; 343 mg sodium.

BROWN RICE RISOTTO WITH BUTTERNUT SQUASH, SHAVED PECORINO, AND GRANNY SMITH APPLE "CAVIAR" GARNISH

SERVES 4

This risotto is made with brown medium-grain rice instead of arborio rice to give it a nuttier taste and added nutrition.

1½ cups medium-grain brown rice

2 tablespoons extra-virgin olive oil

1½ medium yellow onions, finely minced

6 cloves garlic, minced

¾ cup white wine

6 cups low-sodium vegetable broth

½ large butternut squash

1 pinch nutmeg

1 pinch cinnamon

Salt and pepper to taste

1 tablespoon extra-virgin olive oil

2 tablespoons shaved pecorino cheese or Parmesano-Reggiano

For the apple caviar:

3 Granny Smith apples

1 tablespoon fresh lemon juice

To make the risotto: Heat the vegetable stock in a stockpot until simmering. In another pot, heat 1 tablespoon olive oil. Add the onions and garlic, season with salt and pepper, and cook until the onions are translucent.

Add the brown rice and coat it with the onion-garlic mixture. Add the white wine and cook over medium-high heat until the wine has been completely absorbed.

Add 1 ladle of the hot chicken stock at a time, stirring it into the risotto until the rice absorbs the liquid. Repeat this process, stirring the risotto constantly until it is tender but still has a little bite.

To make the butternut squash: Coat the half squash with 1 tablespoon olive oil, nutmeg, cinnamon, and salt and pepper. Place cut side down on a baking sheet lined with foil and bake in a 425°F oven for 25 minutes, until tender and soft. Scoop out the squash flesh and stir it into the finished risotto.

For the apple "caviar," peel the apples and quarter them. Chop into very fine dice and stir in the lemon juice.

Spoon the risotto into serving dishes and garnish with the pecorino cheese and apple "caviar."

PER SERVING (EXCLUDING UNKNOWN ITEMS): 600 calories; 10 g fat (14.9% calories from fat); 26 g protein; 100 g carbohydrate; 13 g dietary fiber; 2 mg cholesterol; 840 mg sodium.

· WHOLE WHEAT RIGATONI WITH OVEN ROASTED · EGGPLANT, MARINARA SAUCE, AND BASIL

SERVES 4

Marinara Sauce:

1 tablespoon extra-virgin olive oil

½ cup minced yellow onion

1 tablespoon chopped fresh parsley

1 clove garlic, peeled and minced

4 cups tomato puree

1 large basil stem, leaves removed

1 teaspoon kosher salt

Eggplant:

1 medium eggplant, cut diagonally
  in thin slices

2 teaspoons extra-virgin olive oil

1 teaspoon minced garlic

1 pound whole wheat pasta, rigatoni
  recommended

To make the marinara sauce: Heat the olive oil in a large nonreactive pot over
  moderate heat. Add the onion and sauté until translucent, about 8 minutes.
  Add the parsley and garlic and cook briefly to release their fragrance. Add
  the tomato puree, basil, and salt.

Simmer briskly until reduced to a saucelike consistency, stirring occasionally
  so nothing sticks to the bottom of the pot. If the sauce thickens too much
  before the flavors have developed, add a little water and continue
  cooking.

Taste and adjust the seasoning. Remove the basil stem before serving.

To make the eggplant: Preheat the oven to 350°F.

Place the eggplants in a baking pan, drizzle with the olive oil, and bake for
  15–20 minutes until tender.

Coarsely chop the eggplant and toss with the minced garlic.

Cook the pasta according to the package directions and drain. Toss the pasta
  with the eggplant and sauce. Divide it evenly among the serving bowls.

PER SERVING (EXCLUDING UNKNOWN ITEMS): 585 calories; 8 g fat (11.2% calories from
fat); 22 g protein; 118 g carbohydrate; 18 g dietary fiber; 0 mg cholesterol; 1481 mg
sodium.

· SOY-GLAZED ROASTED SALMON WITH QUINOA, · CUCUMBER, AND MINT SALAD

SERVES 4

1 cup quinoa (raw whole grain)

2½ cups vegetable stock

2 tablespoons lemon juice

2 tablespoons extra-virgin olive oil

2 cloves garlic, peeled and minced

Salt and pepper to taste

1 cucumber, peeled and sliced

1 red bell pepper, seeded and diced

½ cup minced mint leaves

1 cup low-sodium soy sauce

¼ cup honey

½ teaspoon peeled and minced garlic

1 pound salmon fillet, cut into 4 steaks

To make the salad: Cook the quinoa in the stock, stirring occasionally, until it fluffs up, about 15 minutes. While the quinoa is cooking, whisk together the lemon juice, olive oil, garlic cloves, salt, and pepper to make a dressing. When the quinoa has finished cooking, allow it to cool slightly and toss with the cucumber, bell pepper, mint, and dressing. Refrigerate to cool.

To make the soy glaze: Combine the soy sauce, honey, and minced garlic in a small saucepan. Stir the mixture over medium-high heat until the glaze is reduced by about one-third, about 10 minutes.

Pour one-third of the glaze into a small bowl and set aside. Pour the remainder into a shallow 2- to 3-quart baking dish. Set the salmon pieces in the dish, skin side up, and let marinate for 15 minutes, then turn over.

To make the fish: Bake the salmon in a 450°F oven until the salmon is opaque at the edges but is still translucent in the center, 15 to 20 minutes. Cut to test. Remove from the oven. Set the oven to broil. Brush the salmon with half of the reserved glaze and broil 6 inches from the heat until the salmon steaks are opaque but still moist-looking in the center of the thickest part, about 3 minutes.

PER SERVING (EXCLUDING UNKNOWN ITEMS): 582 calories; 16 g fat (23.9% calories from fat); 37 g protein; 75 g carbohydrate; 7 g dietary fiber; 61 mg cholesterol; 3508 mg sodium.

• WHOLE WHEAT PENNE WITH TUSCAN WHITE • BEAN RAGOUT, ROSEMARY GRILLED SHRIMP, AND SHAVED PARMESAN

SERVES 4

12 ounces whole wheat pasta,
  penne recommended
1 cup cannellini beans, rinsed
  and drained
2 tablespoons extra-virgin olive oil
8 large shrimp, peeled (tail left on)
  and deveined
Salt to taste
3 cloves garlic, peeled and sliced

½ teaspoon red chili flakes
1 medium-size tomato, seeded and
  diced
⅓ cup basil leaves
⅓ cup fresh rosemary
Juice of half a lemon
Pepper to taste
2 tablespoons chopped Italian
  flat-leaf parsley

Cook the penne pasta according to package directions. Drain.

Meanwhile, drain the cannellini beans over a bowl and reserve the liquid. Put the white beans in a large skillet with just enough liquid to moisten them. Add 1 tablespoon olive oil and bring the beans to a low simmer. Keep them warm while you prepare the shrimp.

Heat the remaining 1 tablespoon olive oil in a large skillet over high heat. Add the shrimp, season with salt, and cook about 1 minute, tossing frequently. Remove the shrimp with tongs to a bowl. Add the garlic to the pan and sauté until the garlic browns. Stir in the chili flakes and cook for 1 minute. Add the tomato, basil, and rosemary, stir briefly, and then add the lemon juice. Season with salt and pepper. Cook for about 1 minute and then stir in the shrimp. Toss well and cook briefly to reheat the shrimp. Remove the shrimp mixture to a plate and sprinkle with parsley.

Spoon the cannellini beans on a platter or individual plates and top with the shrimp and pasta. Serve warm.

PER SERVING (EXCLUDING UNKNOWN ITEMS): 550 calories; 9 g fat (13.6% calories from fat); 27 g protein; 97 g carbohydrate; 16 g dietary fiber; 22 mg cholesterol; 45 mg sodium.

SERVES 4

This dish is perfect for anyone who only has time to cook on the weekends. Make enough for a week's worth of dinners at one time or freeze in portions to use later on.

2 tablespoons extra-virgin
  olive oil
1 red onion, peeled and chopped
½ red bell pepper, seeded and diced
½ yellow bell pepper, seeded and
  diced
½ green bell pepper, seeded and
  diced
4 cloves garlic, peeled and minced
Salt and pepper to taste
2 tablespoons chili powder
1 tablespoon cumin
1 tablespoon paprika
6 ounces canned black beans,
  rinsed and drained

6 ounces canned kidney beans, rinsed
  and drained
6 ounces canned pinto beans, rinsed
14 ounces tomato sauce
14 ounces stewed tomatoes
Sachet of 1 cinnamon stick and
  4 bay leaves
½ zucchini, diced
½ yellow squash, diced
1 ear corn, kernels cut off the cob
2 tablespoons minced fresh cilantro
1 jalapeño pepper, seeded and
  minced
4 tablespoons nonfat sour cream

Heat up a pot with olive oil over medium heat. Add the onions, peppers, and garlic, salt and pepper, chili powder, cumin, and paprika. Cook over medium heat for approximately 10 minutes, until the vegetables soften.

Add the canned black, kidney, and pinto beans, tomato sauce, stewed tomatoes, and herb sachet. Simmer uncovered for 30 minutes.

Add the zucchini, yellow squash, and corn. Simmer 5 minutes more. Finish with the cilantro and jalapeños.

Ladle the chili into bowls and garnish with the sour cream.

PER SERVING (EXCLUDING UNKNOWN ITEMS): 314 calories; 9 g fat (24.7% calories from fat); 13 g protein; 51 g carbohydrate; 12 g dietary fiber; 2 mg cholesterol; 1189 mg sodium.

· STEAMED CLAMS WITH WHOLE WHEAT LINGUINE ·
AND BASIL–WHITE WINE SAUCE

SERVES 4

14 ounces whole wheat linguine

2 tablespoons extra-virgin olive oil

4 cloves garlic, chopped

⅓ cup dry white wine

8 ounces canned clams with juice

4 tablespoons chopped fresh basil

2 dozen fresh clams

Salt and pepper

In a large pot of boiling salted water, cook the linguine until tender but still firm to the bite, stirring occasionally. Drain but do not rinse.

While the pasta is cooking, heat the olive oil in a large heavy skillet over medium-high heat. Add the garlic and sauté until fragrant, about 30 seconds. Add the wine and allow to cook about 30 seconds. Add the canned clams with its juice and the basil. Add the fresh clams and cover. Lower the heat to medium and cook until the clams open, about 6 minutes. Using tongs, transfer the fresh clams to a plate. Discard any clams that do not open. Add the cooked pasta to the sauce in the skillet. Toss over medium-high heat until the sauce coats the pasta, about 1 minute. Season to taste with salt and pepper. Divide the pasta among the bowls, top with fresh clams, and serve.

PER SERVING (EXCLUDING UNKNOWN ITEMS): 572 calories; 10 g fat (15.8% calories from fat); 40 g protein; 81 g carbohydrate; 8 g dietary fiber; 68 mg cholesterol; 122 mg sodium.

· SPICY TURKEY-CHIPOTLE MEATLOAF WITH SWEET · POTATO PUREE AND GRILLED VEGETABLES

SERVES 4

Adding oats to the meatloaf mixture adds texture and nutrition. This dish can be made ahead of time and reheated.

⅓ cup quick-cooking oats	2 tablespoons ketchup
¼ cup skim milk	Salt and pepper to taste
1 pound ground turkey	6 ounces tomato sauce
½ medium yellow onion, finely chopped	2 ounces chipotle chilies (canned or fresh)
½ cup green bell pepper, finely chopped	4 medium sweet potatoes
	6 tablespoons chicken stock
1 egg, beaten	8 ounces zucchini, sliced lengthwise
1 teaspoon Worcestershire sauce	½ red bell pepper, sliced lengthwise

Preheat the oven to 350°F. In a large bowl, combine the oats and milk. Add the turkey, chopped onion, red bell pepper, egg, Worcestershire sauce, ketchup, salt, and a few grinds of pepper. Mix until well combined.

Transfer the mixture to a 9 by 13–inch baking dish and shape into a loaf about 5 inches wide and 2½ inches high. In a blender, combine the tomato sauce and chipotle chilies until smooth. Pour the tomato-chipotle sauce over the meatloaf and bake about 1 hour, or until cooked through. Remove from the oven and let rest for 10 to 15 minutes before slicing.

Peel the sweet potatoes and cut into 1-inch pieces. In a small saucepan, boil the potatoes in salted water for 15 minutes or until very tender. Drain well in a colander. In a food processor, puree the potatoes with the chicken stock until smooth. Adjust the salt and pepper if desired.

Prepare a hot grill pan and sear the zucchini and green bell pepper until tender, approximately 3 minutes per side depending on the thickness of the slices.

Serve the meatloaf on top of the sweet potato puree and top with the
zucchini and green bell pepper.

PER SERVING (EXCLUDING UNKNOWN ITEMS): 410 calories; 12 g fat (25.6% calories
from fat); 28 g protein; 49 g carbohydrate; 8 g dietary fiber; 143 mg cholesterol;
758 mg sodium.

· GRILLED CHICKEN PANINI WITH FIGS, ARUGULA, · AND SMOKED GOUDA

SERVES 4

This is a delicious quick meal with lots of protein and a boost of fiber from the multi-grain bread and figs.

4 skinless boneless chicken breasts
Extra-virgin olive oil
¼ teaspoon salt
¼ teaspoon ground black pepper
2 teaspoons chopped fresh rosemary
1 clove fresh garlic, peeled and
   minced

8 dried figs, sliced
8 slices multigrain bread
1 large tomato, sliced
12 pieces arugula, washed and
   patted dry
½ cup thinly sliced smoked Gouda
   cheese

Preheat the grill to medium-high heat.

Brush the chicken with olive oil and season with salt, pepper, rosemary, and garlic.

Place the chicken on a lightly oiled grill grate and cook for 7 minutes per side, or until the juices run clear and the chicken is no longer pink. Remove from grill and allow to cool for 5–10 minutes.

Spread the figs on 4 slices of bread. Place the tomato slices, arugula, cheese, and chicken breasts on the bread.

Cover with the remaining 4 slices, brush with olive oil, and place on the grill. Cook these panini for 4 minutes per side or until the cheese melts. Remove from the heat and serve.

PER SERVING (EXCLUDING UNKNOWN ITEMS): 593 calories; 16 g fat (24.4% calories from fat); 63 g protein; 51 g carbohydrate; 9 g dietary fiber; 159 mg cholesterol; 647 mg sodium.

· GRILLED MAHIMAHI WITH MANGO-BLACK · BEAN SALSA AND BROWN RICE

SERVES 4

For the salsa:

1 large mango, pitted and chopped

⅓ cup chopped green onion

8 ounces canned black beans, rinsed and drained

⅓ cup finely chopped fresh cilantro leaves

¼ cup finely chopped fresh mint leaves

1 jalapeño pepper, seeded and chopped

Juice of 2 limes

Salt

For the rice:

1¼ cups medium-grain brown rice

2½ cups water

For the fish:

2 teaspoons extra-virgin olive oil

1 clove garlic, peeled and minced

1 teaspoon low-sodium soy sauce

1 teaspoon Dijon mustard

4 mahimahi steaks

Salt to taste

To make the salsa: Toss in a bowl the mango, green onion, black beans, cilantro, mint, jalapeño, and juice of 1 lime. Season to taste with salt. Allow to stand at room temperature to allow the flavors to meld.

To make the brown rice: Combine the brown rice and water in a pot with a lid. Season with a small amount of salt if desired. Over high heat, uncovered, bring the water to a boil and then put the lid on the pot and lower the heat to a simmer. Let simmer for 20 minutes, then turn off the heat and let the rice sit in the covered pot for another 15 minutes.

To make the fish: Preheat a grill pan or the broiler of your oven. In a small bowl, whisk the juice of 1 lime, olive oil, garlic, soy sauce, and mustard. Brush the mahimahi steaks with half of this mixture.

Place the mahimahi steaks on the grill and cook to desired temperature, turning only once. Brush the mahimahi steaks once again after turning.

Serve the mahimahi topped with salsa along with the rice.

PER SERVING (EXCLUDING UNKNOWN ITEMS): 581 calories; 13 g fat (20.2% calories from fat); 48 g protein; 67 g carbohydrate; 6 g dietary fiber; 65 mg cholesterol; 319 mg sodium.

• SPANISH PAELLA WITH TURKEY, ARTICHOKES, • PEAS, AND PINE NUTS

SERVES 4

2 teaspoons extra-virgin olive oil

½ large yellow onion, peeled and chopped

1 red bell pepper, seeded and diced

2 cloves garlic, peeled and minced

1 cup frozen artichoke hearts, thawed

1½ tablespoons green olives, chopped

1⅓ cups low-sodium chicken broth

1 cup water

⅔ cup medium-grain brown rice

1 teaspoon salt

½ teaspoon paprika

2 saffron threads (optional)

⅔ cup cooked and chopped boneless skinless turkey breast

⅓ cup frozen green peas, thawed

⅛ cup pine nuts (optional)

Heat the olive oil in a large skillet over medium heat. Add the onion, bell pepper, and garlic, and sauté for 2 minutes. Add the artichoke hearts and olives, and sauté for 2 minutes. Add the broth and water and bring to a boil. Stir in the rice, salt, paprika, and saffron. Cover, lower the heat, and simmer for 25 minutes.

Stir in the turkey, peas, and pine nuts if using. Heat for 5 minutes until the liquid has been absorbed and the peas are heated through.

Remove from the heat and let stand covered for 5 minutes. Fluff with a fork and serve.

PER SERVING (EXCLUDING UNKNOWN ITEMS): 248 calories; 5 g fat (18.4% calories from fat); 15 g protein; 35 g carbohydrate; 6 g dietary fiber; 18 mg cholesterol; 743 mg sodium.

• MARINATED SKIRT STEAK WITH CHIMICHURRI AND • SALSA VERDE SAUCES

SERVES 4

Chimichurri Sauce:

⅔ cup sherry vinegar

2 tablespoons lemon juice

1 cup Italian flat-leaf parsley, minced

4 tablespoons basil leaves, minced

1 tablespoon fresh oregano, minced

3 tablespoons garlic, peeled and minced

2 tablespoons shallots, peeled and minced

¼ teaspoon ground black pepper

½ teaspoon salt

¼ teaspoon crushed red pepper flakes

½ cup extra-virgin olive oil

Salsa Verde:

2 large chili peppers

8 ounces tomatillos, husked, rinsed, and diced

1½ cups low-sodium chicken broth

2 large green onions, chopped

1 large serrano chili, stemmed and seeded

1 clove garlic

½ cup fresh cilantro leaves

Salt to taste

1 tablespoon fresh lime juice

Skirt Steak:

1 pound skirt steak

Salt and pepper to taste

To make the Chimichurri sauce: In the bowl of a food processor, combine the sherry vinegar, lemon juice, parsley, basil, oregano, garlic, shallots, and olive oil. Pulse until well blended but do not puree.

Add the black pepper, salt, and crushed red pepper.

Transfer the sauce to a nonreactive bowl, cover with plastic wrap, and set at room temperature.

To make the salsa verde: Blacken the chilies on all sides directly over a gas flame or in a broiler. Place in a paper bag and let stand for 10 minutes so the skin steams loose. Peel, seed, and chop the chilies.

Combine the tomatillos, broth, green onions, serrano chili, and garlic in a medium saucepan. Bring to a boil over medium-high heat. Reduce the heat to medium-low and simmer until the mixture is reduced to 1⅔ cups, stirring occasionally, about 18 minutes.

Transfer the mixture to a blender and add the chopped chilies and cilantro. Puree until smooth.

Season the salsa with salt and add lime juice. Cover with plastic wrap and set aside at room temperature.

To make the steak: Season the steak with salt and pepper.

Preheat a grill to medium heat. Cook for 6 minutes on the first side, then rotate the steak 45 degrees. Cook 6 minutes more. Turn the steak over and continue to cook until the steak is done, 6 to 8 minutes for medium-rare.

Once cooked, lay the steak on a clean cutting board and allow it to rest for 5 to 7 minutes before slicing across the grain into 2-inch-wide strips.

Serve the skirt steak with chimichurri and salsa verde sauce.

PER SERVING (EXCLUDING UNKNOWN ITEMS): 522 calories; 40 g fat (66.8% calories from fat); 29 g protein; 16 g carbohydrate; 3 g dietary fiber; 58 mg cholesterol; 1464 mg sodium.

APPENDIX

BODY MASS INDEX (*BMI*)

Height	18	19	20	21	22	23	24	25	26	27	28	29	30	31	32	33	34	35	36	37	38	39	40
										Body Weight (pounds)													
4'10"	86	91	96	100	105	110	115	119	124	129	134	138	143	148	153	158	162	167	172	177	181	186	191
4'11"	89	94	99	104	109	114	119	124	128	133	138	143	148	153	158	163	168	173	178	183	188	193	198
5'0"	92	97	102	107	112	118	123	128	133	138	143	148	153	158	163	168	174	179	184	189	194	199	204
5'1"	95	100	106	111	116	122	127	132	137	143	148	153	158	164	169	174	180	185	190	195	201	206	211
5'2"	98	104	109	115	120	126	131	136	142	147	153	158	164	169	175	180	186	191	196	202	207	213	218
5'3"	102	107	113	118	124	130	135	141	146	152	158	163	169	175	180	186	191	197	203	208	214	220	225
5'4"	105	110	116	122	128	134	140	145	151	157	163	169	174	180	186	192	197	204	209	215	221	227	232
5'5"	108	114	120	126	132	138	144	150	156	162	168	174	180	186	192	198	204	210	216	222	228	234	240
5'6"	112	118	124	130	136	142	148	155	161	167	173	179	186	192	198	204	210	216	223	229	235	241	247
5'7"	115	121	127	134	140	146	153	159	166	172	178	185	191	198	204	211	217	223	230	236	242	249	255
5'8"	118	125	131	138	144	151	158	165	171	177	184	190	197	203	210	216	223	230	236	243	249	256	262
5'9"	122	128	135	142	149	155	162	169	176	182	189	196	203	209	216	223	230	236	243	250	257	263	270
5'10"	126	132	139	146	153	160	167	174	181	188	195	202	209	216	222	229	236	243	250	257	264	271	278
5'11"	129	136	143	150	157	165	172	179	186	193	200	208	215	222	229	236	243	250	257	265	272	279	286
6'0"	132	140	147	154	162	169	177	184	191	199	206	213	221	228	235	242	250	258	265	272	279	287	294
6'1"	136	144	151	159	166	174	182	189	197	204	212	219	227	235	242	250	257	265	272	280	288	295	302
6'2"	141	148	155	163	171	179	186	194	202	210	218	225	233	241	249	256	264	272	280	287	295	303	311
6'3"	144	152	160	168	176	184	192	200	208	216	224	232	240	248	256	264	272	279	287	295	303	311	319
6'4"	148	156	164	172	180	189	197	205	213	221	230	238	246	254	263	271	279	287	295	304	312	320	328
6'5"	151	160	168	176	185	193	202	210	218	227	235	244	252	261	269	277	286	294	303	311	319	328	336
6'6"	155	164	172	181	190	198	207	216	224	233	241	250	259	267	276	284	293	302	310	319	328	336	345

UNDERWEIGHT	HEALTHY WEIGHT	OVERWEIGHT	OBESE
(<18.5)	(18.5–24.9)	(25–29.9)	(≥30)

Find your height along the left-hand column and look across the row until you find the number that is closest to your weight. The number at the top of that column identifies your BMI.

From A. Must, G. E. Dallal, and W. H. Dietz, "Reference Data for Obesity: 85th and 95th Percentiles of Body Mass Index (wt/ht^2) and Triceps Skinfold Thickness." *American Journal of Clinical Nutrition* 53 (1991): 839–846. Adapted with permission by the *American Journal of Clinical Nutrition*, © *American Journal of Clinical Nutrition*, American Society for Clinical Nutrition.

FIBER CONTENT OF FOODS

To consume more fiber, eat more whole fruits and vegetables, whole grains, and beans. Nuts are also rich in fiber, but they are energy dense, so eat them in small amounts. Use the following list to guide your food choices. It is adapted from research conducted by the Tufts University School of Medicine in Boston and published in the *Tufts Health & Nutrition Letter*.

FRUITS*	GRAMS OF FIBER
Apple (with skin)	4
Banana	3
Blueberries, ½ cup	2
Cantaloupe, 1 cup diced	1
Dates, ⅛ cup dry, chopped	2
Grapefruit, ½	2
Grapes, 1 cup	2
Nectarine (with skin)	2
Orange	3
Peach (with skin)	2
Pear (with skin)	4
Plum (with skin)	1
Prunes (dried), 10	2
Raisins, ⅛ cup	1
Raspberries, ½ cup	4
Strawberries, ½ cup	2
Watermelon, 1 cup diced	1

VEGETABLES†	GRAMS OF FIBER
Broccoli, ½ cup cooked, chopped	2
Broccoli, ½ cup chopped	1

*All values are for 1 medium-size fruit unless otherwise indicated.

†All values are for raw, uncooked vegetables unless otherwise indicated.

HOW TO READ A FOOD LABEL

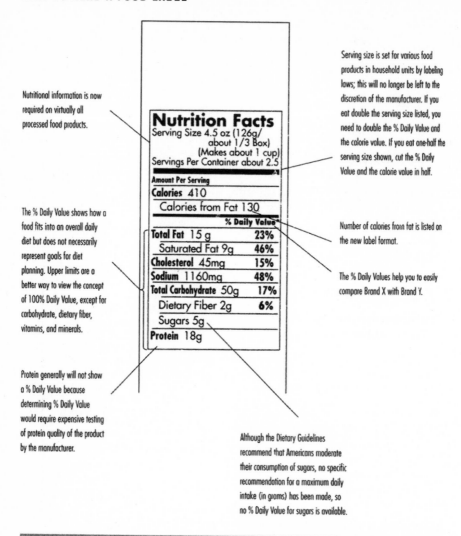

Nutritional information is now required on virtually all processed food products.

The % Daily Value shows how a food fits into an overall daily diet but does not necessarily represent goals for diet planning. Upper limits are a better way to view the concept of 100% Daily Value, except for carbohydrate, dietary fiber, vitamins, and minerals.

Protein generally will not show a % Daily Value because determining % Daily Value would require expensive testing of protein quality of the product by the manufacturer.

Nutrition Facts
Serving Size 4.5 oz (126g/
about 1/3 Box)
(Makes about 1 cup)
Servings Per Container about 2.5

Amount Per Serving

Calories 410
Calories from Fat 130

% Daily Value*

Total Fat 15 g	23%
Saturated Fat 9g	46%
Cholesterol 45mg	15%
Sodium 1160mg	48%
Total Carbohydrate 50g	17%
Dietary Fiber 2g	6%
Sugars 5g	
Protein 18g	

Serving size is set for various food products in household units by labeling laws; this will no longer be left to the discretion of the manufacturer. If you eat double the serving size listed, you need to double the % Daily Value and the calorie value. If you eat one-half the serving size shown, cut the % Daily Value and the calorie value in half.

Number of calories from fat is listed on the new label format.

The % Daily Values help you to easily compare Brand X with Brand Y.

Although the Dietary Guidelines recommend that Americans moderate their consumption of sugars, no specific recommendation for a maximum daily intake (in grams) has been made, so no % Daily Value for sugars is available.

The Nutrition Facts panel on a current food label. The box is broken into two parts: A is the top, and B is the bottom. The % Daily Value listed on the label is the percentage of the generally accepted amount of a nutrient needed daily that is present in 1 serving of the product. You can use the % Daily Values to compare your diet with current nutrition recommendations for certain diet components. Let's consider dietary fiber. Assume that you consume 2,000 kcal. per day, which is the energy intake corresponding to the % Daily Values listed on labels. If the total % Daily Value for dietary fiber in all the foods you eat in one day adds up to 100%, your diet meets the recommendations for dietary fiber.

218 | THE 4 DAY DIET

Many vitamin and mineral amounts no longer need to be listed on the nutrition label. Only Vitamin A, Vitamin C, calcium, and iron remain. The interest in or risk of deficiencies of the other vitamins and minerals is deemed too low to warrant inclusion.

Some % Daily Value standards, such as grams of total fat, increase as energy intake increases. The % Daily Values on the label are based on a 2,000-kcal. diet. This is important to note if you don't consume at least 2,000 kcal. per day.

Labels on larger packages may list the number of calories per gram of fat, carbohydrate, and protein.

Ingredients, listed in descending order by weight, will appear here or in another place on the package. The sources of some ingredients, such as certain flavorings, will be stated by name to help people better identify ingredients that they avoid for health, religious, or other reasons.

Vitamin A 10% • Vitamin C 0%
Calcium 30% • Iron 15%

Percent Daily Values are based on a 2,000 calorie diet. Your daily values may be higher or lower depending on your calorie needs:

		Calories:	2,000	2,500
Total Fat	Less than		65g	80g
Sat Fat	Less than		20g	25g
Cholest	Less than		300mg	300mg
Sodium	Less than		2,400mg	2,400mg
Total Carb			300g	375g
Fiber			25g	30g

Calories per gram:
Fat 9 • Carbohydrate 4
• Protein 4

INGREDIENTS: WATER, ENRICHED MACARONI [ENRICHED FLOUR [NIACIN, FERROUS SULFATE (IRON), THIAMINE MONONITRATE AND RIBOFLAVIN], EGG WHITE), FLOUR, CHEDDAR CHEESE (MILK, CHEESE CULTURE, SALT, ENZYME), SPICES, MARGARINE (PARTIALLY HYDROGENATED SOYBEAN OIL, WATER, SOY LECITHIN, MONO- AND DIGLYCERIDES, BETA CARO- TENE FOR COLOR, VITAMIN A PALMITATE), AND MALTODEXTRIN.

Source: Wardlaw, Gordon M., *Contemporary Nutrition*, 4th ed. (New York: McGraw Hill Companies, Inc., 2000).

CALORIC EXPENDITURE
DURING VARIOUS ACTIVITIES

ACTIVITY	CAL/MIN*
Sleeping	1.2
Resting in bed	1.3
Sitting, normally	1.3
Sitting, reading	1.3
Lying, quietly	1.3
Sitting, eating	1.5
Sitting, playing cards	1.5
Standing, normally	1.5
Classwork, lecture (listening)	1.7
Conversing	1.8
Personal toilet	2.0
Sitting, writing	2.6
Standing, light activity	2.6
Washing and dressing	2.6
Washing and shaving	2.6
Driving a car	2.8
Washing clothes	3.1
Walking indoors	3.1
Shining shoes	3.2
Making bed	3.4
Dressing	3.4
Showering	3.4
Driving motorcycle	3.4

*Depends on efficiency and body size. Add 10 percent for each 15 lb. over 150; subtract 10 percent for each 15 lb. under 150.

ACTIVITY	CAL/MIN
Metalworking	3.5
House painting	3.5
Cleaning windows	3.7
Carpentry	3.8
Farming chores	3.8
Sweeping floors	3.9
Plastering walls	4.1
Repairing trucks and automobiles	4.2
Ironing clothes	4.2
Farming, planting, hoeing, raking	4.7
Mixing cement	4.7
Mopping floors	4.9
Repaving roads	5.0
Gardening, weeding	5.6
Stacking lumber	5.8
Sawing with chain saw	6.2
Working with stone, masonry	6.3
Working with pick and shovel	6.7
Farming, haying, plowing with horse	6.7
Shoveling (miners)	6.8
Shoveling snow	7.5
Walking down stairs	7.1
Chopping wood	7.5
Sawing with crosscut saw	7.5–10.5
Tree felling (ax)	8.4–12.7
Gardening, digging	8.6
Walking up stairs	10.0–18.0
Playing pool or billiards	1.8
Canoeing, 2.5 mph–4.0 mph	3.0–7.0

ACTIVITY	CAL/MIN
Playing volleyball, recreational to competitive	3.5–8.0
Golfing, foursome to twosome	3.7–5.0
Pitching horseshoes	3.8
Playing baseball (except pitcher)	4.7
Playing Ping-Pong or table tennis	4.9–7.0
Practicing calisthenics	5.0
Rowing, pleasure to vigorous	5.0–15.0
Cycling, easy to hard	5.0–15.0
Skating, recreational to vigorous	5.0–15.0
Practicing archery	5.2
Playing badminton, recreational to competitive	5.2–10.0
Playing basketball, half or full court (more for fast break)	6.0–9.0
Bowling (while active)	7.0
Playing tennis, recreational to competitive	7.0–11.0
Waterskiing	8.0
Playing soccer	9.0
Snowshoeing (2.5 mph)	9.0
Slide board	9.0–13.0
Playing handball or squash	10.0
Mountain climbing	10.0–15.0
Skipping rope	10.0–15.0
Practicing judo or karate	13.0
Playing football (while active)	13.3
Wrestling	14.4
Skiing	
Moderate to steep	8.0–20.0

ACTIVITY	CAL/MIN
Downhill racing	16.5
Cross-country; 3–10 mph	9.0–20.0
Swimming	
Leisurely	6.0
Crawl, 25–50 yd/min.	6.0–12.5
Butterfly, 50 yd/min.	14.0
Backstroke, 25–50 yd/min.	6.0–12.5
Breaststroke, 25–50 yd/min.	6.0–12.5
Sidestroke, 40 yd/min.	11.0
Dancing	
Modern, moderate to vigorous	4.2–5.7
Ballroom, waltz to rumba	5.7–7.0
Square	7.7
Walking	
Road or field (3.5 mph)	5.6–7.0
Snow, hard to soft (2.5–3.5 mph)	10.0–20.0
Uphill, 15 percent grade (3.5 mph)	8.0–15.0
Downhill, 5–10 percent grade (2.5 mph)	3.5–3.7
15–20 percent grade (2.5 mph)	3.7–4.3
Hiking, 40-lb. pack (3.0 mph)	6.8
Running	
12-min. mile (5 mph)	10.0
8-min. mile (7.5 mph)	15.0
6-min. mile (10 mph)	20.0
5-min. mile (12 mph)	25.0

Source: Sharkey, Brian J., PhD., *Fitness and Health*, 4th ed. (Champaign: Human Kinetics, 1997).

INDEX

Note: "t" in a page number means "table."

beef
   Beef Satay Skewers with Peanut Dip-
      ping Sauce, 187
   ground, substitution for, 90t
   Marinated Skirt Steak with
      Chimichurri and Salsa Verde
      Sauces, 213
   in modular eating plans, 140
   roast, 140
behavioral changes, rewarding yourself
   for, 95–96
berries, in modular eating plans, 108,
   113, 140, 141
bicycling, calories burned, 77t
"big person" habits, 66–67
black beans, 109
black-eyed peas, 109
blood pressure
   high, obesity and, 4t
   lower, as weight program goal, 20
blood sugars
   glycemic index related to, 44–46
   insulin as stabilizing, 28
blueberries
   fiber in, 58t, 217t
   in modular eating plans, 113, 140,
      141
body
   analogy with a car, 82–83
   control of, by the mind, in sports,
      61–63
   keeping it off-kilter with a variety of
      foods, 97–98
body fat measurements
   vs. BMI, 5
   inaccuracy of, 17
body image, your assessing it, 7–9
   having a false picture of, 8, 64–65
   self quiz for, 8–9
Body Mass Index (BMI), 3–4
   how to calculate, 3–4t, 216t
   as objective measure, 5
   setting a new one as goal, 23
bowling, calories burned, 77t
Bradley, Bill, 1–2
brain
   reward system of the, 50–51
   training it to resist temptation, 50–54
bran, 117
   fiber in, 58t

bran cereal, 117
   glycemic index of, 48t
   in modular eating plans, 141
bread
   glycemic index of, 47t
   in modular eating plans, 139
   raisin, 139
   whole wheat, fiber in, 58t
bread pudding, Nutty Oatmeal and
      Whole Wheat Breakfast Bread
      Pudding, 160
breakfast
   amount to eat at, 83–85
   Asian Breakfast Stir-Fry with Soba
      Noodles and Fresh Vegetables, 150
   Country Breakfast Turkey Patty with
      Oatmeal and Side of Fruit, 154
   recipes, 145–64
breast cancer, obesity and, 4t
broad beans, 109
broccoli, fiber in, 217t
buffalo wings, in modular eating plans,
   130
bulgur, fiber in, 58t
burrito
   Breakfast Burrito with Scrambled Egg
      Whites, Pinto Beans, Salsa, and
      Turkey Sausage, 151
   Egg White and Turkey Bacon Break-
      fast Burrito with Pineapple Salsa, 156

café latte, substitution for, 90t
calico beans, 109
calorie expenditure
   with exercise, 75, 77t, 220–223t
   for various activities, 220–223t
calorie intake
   distributing it evenly throughout the
      day, 28
   severely restricted, danger of, 17–18
cancer, obesity and, 4t
candy bar, substitution for, 90t
cannellini beans, 109
canoeing, calories burned, 77t
cantaloupe
   fiber in, 217t
   in modular eating plans, 140
carb loading, 110
cardiovascular exercise
   action of, in weight loss, 76

cottage cheese, in modular eating plans, 91t, 139, 140, 141
couscous, fiber in, 58t
crackers
    glycemic index of, 47t
    in modular eating plans, 140, 141
cravings
    cost-benefit analysis of yielding to, 54
    lack of balance in diet and, 57
    overcoming, by keeping busy, 58–59
    reasons for, 51, 57
    satisfying them in moderation, 56–57
cream, substitution for, 91t
cream cheese
    in modular eating plans, 140
    substitution for, 90t
cream of chicken soup, substitution for, 90t
cream of chicken soup, substitution for, 90t
cream of rice, 117
cream of wheat, 117
cucumbers
    fiber in, 58t
    in modular eating plans, 108, 125, 127, 135

dancing, calories burned, 77t
dates
    fiber in, 217t
    glycemic index of, 47t
Davis, Adele, 85
detox, 107
diabetes, type 2, obesity and, 4t
diet. See food
dieting. See weight-loss program
dinner
    amount to eat at, 85
    recipes, 185–214
directional thought, 61
disappointment, sticking with a weight-loss program despite, 41–42
diseases, related to obesity, 4t
dopamine, 50–51
doughnut, glycemic index of, 47t
dressing, salad
    in modular eating plans, 107, 108, 139
    substitution for, 90t
dyslipidemia, obesity and, 4t

eating
    emotional reasons for, 81, 86–89
    every bite counts, 81–92
    in France vs. in America, 27–28
    making a consumption chart of your daily pattern, 83
    mindful and mindless, 81, 87
    at the right times of day, 83–85
    schedule of, 29, 81
edamame, 109
    in modular eating plans, 139
eggs
    Curried Eggs Benedict with Whole Wheat English Muffins, 155
    in modular eating plans, 103, 111, 113, 125, 127
    Poached Egg with Turkey Bacon, Grilled Tomato, and Black Beans, 163
    Southwestern Baked Eggs, 164
80–20 rule of healthy to unhealthy foods, 51–52
emotional eating, 81, 87–89
emotions
    coping with, other than with food, 88
    and motivation to lose weight, 38
endometrial cancer, obesity and, 4t
endorphins, exercise and, 88
English muffin, in modular eating plans, 90t
ethnic women, believing that BMI doesn't apply to them, 5
exercise
    calorie expenditures for various types of, 77t, 220–223t
    emotional eating avoided by, 88
    and endorphins, 88
    five times a week, as weight program goal, 20
    fun types of, 104
    getting past the discomfort of, 34
    how to start, 76
    in modular eating plans, 107, 108, 111, 113, 114, 115, 124, 125, 127
    need for, while dieting, 75–80
    physical benefits of, 75–76, 78
    seven-day program of, at start of weight loss program, 79t
    types and techniques of, 76–78

meatloaf, Spicy Turkey-Chipotle Meatloaf with Sweet Potato Puree and
Grilled Vegetables, 207
Melba toast, in modular eating plans,
141
metabolism
boosted with resistance exercise, 78
low, during sleep, and weight gain,
85
milestones
aiming for, when attempting big goals,
19
fear of, 68
milk
with breakfast cereal, 117
evaporated, 91t
glycemic index of, 48t
in modular eating plans, 90t, 91t
skim, 48t, 90t
whole, 90t
mind, training it to resist temptation,
49–50
mind-body connection, 61
mind-body disconnect, 66
mindful eating, 87
mindless eating, 81
mirror, loving yourself in, as weight program goal, 20
modular eating plans, 97–137
composed of smaller modules, 97
Induction module, 98–106
Pace module, 128–32
Protein Stretch module, 110–11
Push module, 123–27
Smooth module, 112–16
Transition module, 107–8
variety in, 108, 111
Vigorous module, 133–37
mood, keeping track of, in weight-loss
journal, 9
motivation, 31–48
different for each individual, 31–32
finding your own, 32–36
four questions to ask yourself, 32–35,
45t
typical motivators for starting a weight-
loss program, 37–41
motivation table, 46t
how to prepare, and example of one,
42–44

mozzarella cheese, in modular eating
plans, 90t
muesli, Homemade Muesli and Yogurt
Parfait, 158
mung beans, 109
Murphy, Dan, 61–62
muscle, weight of, 78
muscle-bound appearance, 76
muse, your (a person you admire), as motivation, 34–35
mustard, in modular eating plans, 90t

nachos, substitution for, 91t
Nature's Path breakfast cereals, 121
navy beans, 109
nectarine, fiber in, 217t
negativity, shutting out, 35
New Morning breakfast cereals, 121
Nicklaus, Jack, 71
noodles, in modular eating plans, 140
normal weight, definition of, 4t, 216t
nuts, fiber in, 58t

oat bran, 117
fiber in, 58t
oatmeal, 117
fiber in, 58t
Steel-Cut Oatmeal with Apples, Almonds, and Dates, 147
obesity
definition of, 4t, 216t
health problems related to, 4t
stigma attached to, 41
visual appearance masking, 5
omelet
California Omelet with Egg Whites,
Artichokes, Avocado, and Jack
Cheese, 153
Egg White Omelet with Basil Pesto
and Fresh Fruit, 157
in modular eating plans, 130, 136
Western Omelet with Turkey Ham and
Bell Peppers, 159
orange
fiber in, 217t
glycemic index of, 47t
in modular eating plans, 115, 126, 139
orange juice, frozen, in modular eating
plans, 140
osteoarthrities, obesity and, 4t

overweight
    continuing to act as if one is, even after weight loss, 66–67
    dangers of being, 37–38
    definition of, 4t, 216t
    not looking overweight, 5
    reasons for becoming, 6
    self-image of, as imprisoning, 63–65
oyster sauce, in modular eating plans, 90t

Pace module, 128–32
pacing, by runners, 128
paella, Spanish Paella with Turkey, Artichokes, Peas, and Pine Nuts, 212
pancakes
    Apple and Almond Whole Wheat pancakes, 149
    glycemic index of, 47t
    in modular eating plans, 116, 131
    Whole Wheat Pancakes with Low-Calorie Syrup and Fresh Berries, 145
pancreas, 46
panini, in modular eating plans, 113
parties, tempting food at, 55
pasta
    in modular eating plans, 113, 116
    Whole Wheat Penne with Tuscan White Bean Ragout, Rosemary Grilled Shrimp, and Shaved Parmesan, 204
    Whole Wheat Rigatoni with Oven Roasted Eggplant, Marinara Sauce, and Basil, 202
Patzer, Bryan, 62
peach
    fiber in, 217t
    in modular eating plans, 141
peanut butter, in modular eating plans, 90t, 139, 140, 141
peanuts, glycemic index of, 48t
pear
    fiber in, 58t, 217t
    glycemic index of, 47t
    in modular eating plans, 108, 114, 126, 127, 135
peas, dried, fiber in, 58t

pedometer, 116, 125, 126, 132
peer pressure, as motivator to lose weight, 39
Peking/hoisin sauce, substitution for, 90t
Pepperidge Farm Goldfish Crackers, in modular eating plans, 140
peppers, Stuffed Sweet Peppers with Chicken and Tomatoes, 165
perfection, striving for, as setup for failure, 88
Performance Media, 72
pickle, in modular eating plans, 139
pineapple, in modular eating plans, 91t
pinto beans, 109
pizza
    in modular eating plans, 113
    no-cheese, as substitute for other foods, 91t
    Whole Wheat Neapolitan-Style Pizza with Homemade Tomato Sauce, Turkey Sausage, and Fresh Mozzarella, 190
plateau, not being discouraged when on a, 41
pleasure, brain hormones and, 50–51
plum, fiber in, 217t
popcorn
    air-popped, 90t, 139
    buttered, 90t
    in modular eating plans, 90t, 139
Pop-Tart, substitution for, 90t
positives, focusing on, 65
positive thinking, 35–36
Post breakfast cereals, 121–22
potato, baked, glycemic index of, 47t
potato chips
    baked, 90t
    substitution for, 90t
poultry, protein in, 110
Proper Preparation Prevents Poor Performance (five P's), 55, 123
protein
    daily requirement, 110
    sources of, 110
Protein Stretch module, 110–11
prunes, fiber in, 217t
psyllium, 102
    husk, in modular eating plans, 100, 104
pudding

weight
 attainable and unattainable, 17–18
 definition of underweight, normal,
  overweight, and obese, 4t
 "good" (muscle) vs. "bad" (fat), 78
weight gain, average, per year, among
  Americans, 14–15
weight loss
 physical process of, and body changes,
  17
 time needed to achieve a given goal,
  23–27
 too rapid, 14–15
 weekly pounds of, setting a goal for,
  23–27
weight-loss program
 disappointment with, 64, 66–71
 getting a sense of where you are starting from, 1–11
 having several goals in, not just pounds
  lost, 20
 journal used in, 9–10
 measures of progress in (not just
  pounds), 16–17
 motivation to start one, 36–41
 pools and prizes as motivators, 39
 questions to answer before starting, 2
 realistic goals in, 14–15
 reasons for embarking on one, 31–32,
  36–37
 sticking with, 41–42

weight-loss TV shows, 21–22, 39
Western science, on the mind-body connection, 61
wheat bran, 58t, 117
wheat hearts, 117
wheat Thin crackers, 140
whipped topping, in modular eating
  plans, 139
white beans, 109
white wine sauce, in modular eating
  plans, 91t
will, power of, 62–63
winner, thinking like a, 61–63
Woods, Tiger, 71–72
work boxes, 11t, 45t, 59t, 74t, 92
workplace, tempting foods in the, 55

yogurt
 frozen, 91t
 in modular eating plans, 91t, 100, 104,
  114, 129, 132, 134, 135, 137, 139,
  140
 Yogurt with Granola, Mangoes, and
  Crystallized Ginger, 148
Yoplait Light Smoothie, 140
yo-yo dieting, 21

zucchini
 fiber in, 58t
 Grilled Globe Zucchini "Steak" with
  Quinoa, 180